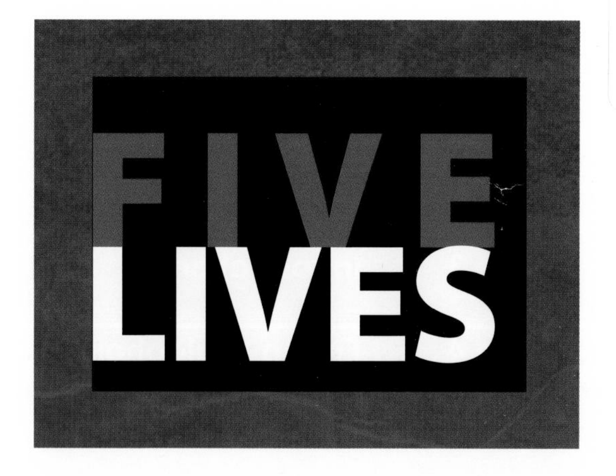

Written by: Kate Davies, Emma Mackinnon, Emma Silvano, Hannah Fletcher and Anna Maria

Tutor and editor: Fiona Prideaux

Editor: Clare Eastland

Designer: Daniel Loveday
www.danielloveday creativesolutions.com

First published 2013 by Southgate Publishers Ltd.

Southgate Publishers Ltd, The Square, Sandford, Crediton, Devon EX17 4LW.

Printed and bound in Great Britain by Brightsea Press, Exeter.

British Library Cataloguing Publication Data.

A CIP catalogue record for this book is available from the British Library.

ISBN 9 781857 411584

Contents

Acknowledgements

The authors would like to thank Fiona Prideaux for encouraging them to write this book, and for her boundless faith in them. Fiona is a wonderful teacher who isn't afraid to take a risk! They thank her for giving them the opportunity to become published writers.

Fiona would like to thank her husband **Jonathan** for his support and encouragement from the very beginning. She couldn't have done it without him.

Emma S would like to thank her Mum and Dad for encouraging her to write and **Anna** would like to thank her two friends for giving her the support and courage to change her life. You truly saved her.

And to **all the family members, friends and colleagues** who have helped the authors along the way. Thank you. Thank you. Thank you!

The authors would like to thank **Devon Adult and Community Learning** for providing the literacy courses along with their inspirational tutor, Fiona. Thank you also to the DACL Community Development Co-ordinator for Exeter, **Lizzie Bond,** for her invaluable help and advice.

The Esther Community is a hostel in Exeter for homeless women and girls with high support and complex needs. It is managed overall by Keychange Charity.

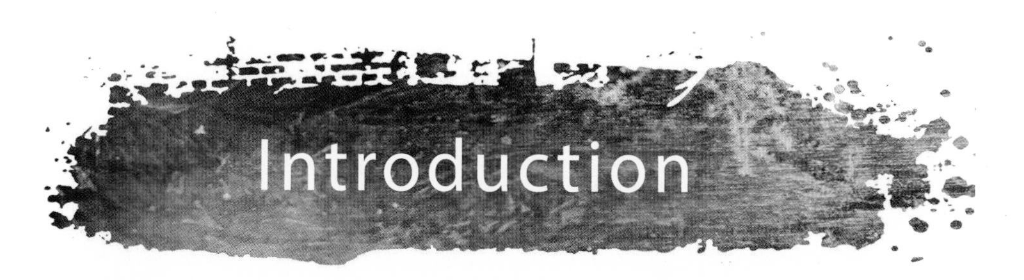

Introduction

This book is about five extraordinary women: Cat, Emma S, Anna, Hannah and Emma M. They have written short autobiographical stories: snapshots of their lives, snapshots that tell the stories of their personal battles through drug and alcohol addiction, domestic violence, self-harming and homelessness. The stories are gritty, honest, humbling and inspiring. They are also a window into a part of society that is often looked down upon and judged. This book gives you an insight into those five lives and, we hope, a greater understanding of them and others like them.

The five met when they were living in a hostel for homeless women in Exeter: The Esther Community. They started a course to improve their literacy and were encouraged to write some autobiographical stories. But it soon became much more than just writing stories.

The women found that the process of writing about their lives helped them to address some of the problems that they had experienced in the past. Writing became a kind of therapy, and once they started they wanted to do more and more.

This book has also been about teamwork and friendship. As the group started writing their autobiographical pieces, they got to know each other much better and, through working together and reading each other's stories, they gained a greater understanding and respect for each other. The friendships that have grown and developed between them have been one of the most positive results of this whole journey.

But more than anything else this book is an example of what can be achieved when expectations are high and when the people working with you believe in you. Writing this book and putting it all together has been an amazing collaborative experience. During the publication process, the authors worked in partnership with the publishers to make editorial, design and marketing decisions. They became part of the team. Their decisions have formed this book and they have made it their own. I would particularly like to thank Rachel and Drummond Johnstone from Southgate for believing in us and making the dream a reality. Huge thanks must also go to our wonderful editor Clare Eastland for her wisdom and guidance, our fabulous illustrator Jemma Cholawo, for putting into pictures what words cannot say, and our brilliant designer Daniel Loveday, especially for his stunning work with the photographs.

This has also been a phenomenal journey for me, their literacy tutor. I feel privileged to have worked with such an inspiring and vibrant group. I have learnt so much from them, and I have immense admiration for their spirit and determination.

We hope that by sharing these stories we will empower others and inspire them to write their own stories.

Fiona Prideaux, Literacy Tutor

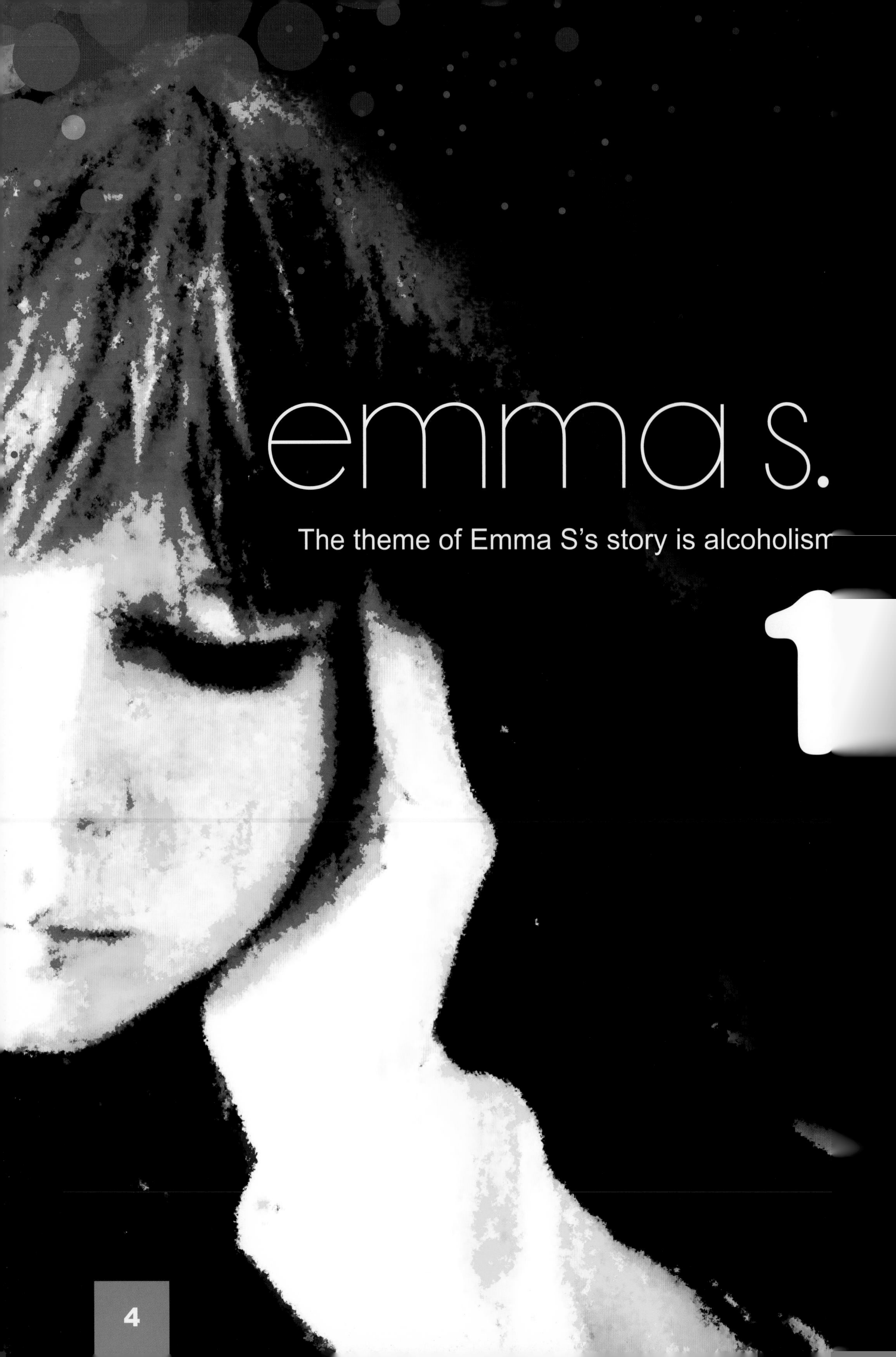

emma s.

The theme of Emma S's story is alcoholism

1

my story

I had a happy childhood, but I was a shy, quiet child and, as the eldest of two, quite overprotected by my parents. I lacked confidence and belief in myself.

When I was sixteen I discovered alcohol and realised that my inhibitions vanished after a glass or two of wine. I became a confident person. Unfortunately my drinking soon escalated out of control and I became an alcoholic. I was an alcoholic for eighteen years. During that time I worked sporadically, begged on the streets in London and Bristol and did anything I could to feed my addiction.

I went into rehab twice but relapsed both times. Finally, aged thirty-four, I had a serious wake-up call from my GP who told me I was dying from alcoholism and had only about four months to live. I took the warning to heart and knew I had to stop drinking or die.

I have been sober for eight years. Life has not all been rosy since then and unfortunately, due to financial problems, I became homeless again. But, in July 2012, I gained a place at a women's hostel where I received amazing support and plentiful opportunities to once again become an accepted member of society. I remain sober as a recovering alcoholic.

I aspire to be a published author and to work as a counsellor within the field of alcohol abuse and recovery.

Teenager

October 1987

The mirror crashed at the bottom of the stairs, smashing into pieces with the force of my throwing it. My mother had managed to dodge out of the way but I could see sparkles of glass shining against the navy blue of her smart, business suit. Her eyes shone up at me, terrified.

Through my alcohol-induced stupor I felt a flash of pain – 'She's scared of me'.

Deep down I knew that I'd done this awful thing because no one seemed to comprehend what was going on in my head, no one seemed to realise the muddle that my mind was in.

I retreated back to my room where a bottle of white wine was sitting on the floor next to a giant stuffed polar bear. I greedily glugged from the bottle as I heard Mum's sobs coming from downstairs.

'Shut up, shut up,' I said silently in my head.

But other thoughts soon took over, 'Where would I get another bottle before college at 4.00 pm?'

All I wanted, needed, was another drink.

I knew I'd have to leave soon if I was to fit in everything that I wanted to do. I needed, after all, to obtain more alcohol as well as consume more, before my afternoon lecture.

I heard the front door closing as Mum left the house to return to work. I drained the wine bottle and knew that I needed another drink, QUICKLY, to attempt to erase the image of Mum's terrified face from my mind. Half stumbling, I grappled with books, paper, a bag, not really paying much attention to which books and notes I was actually grabbing.

My fuzzy brain managed somehow to direct my legs down the stairs and into the lounge. Picking

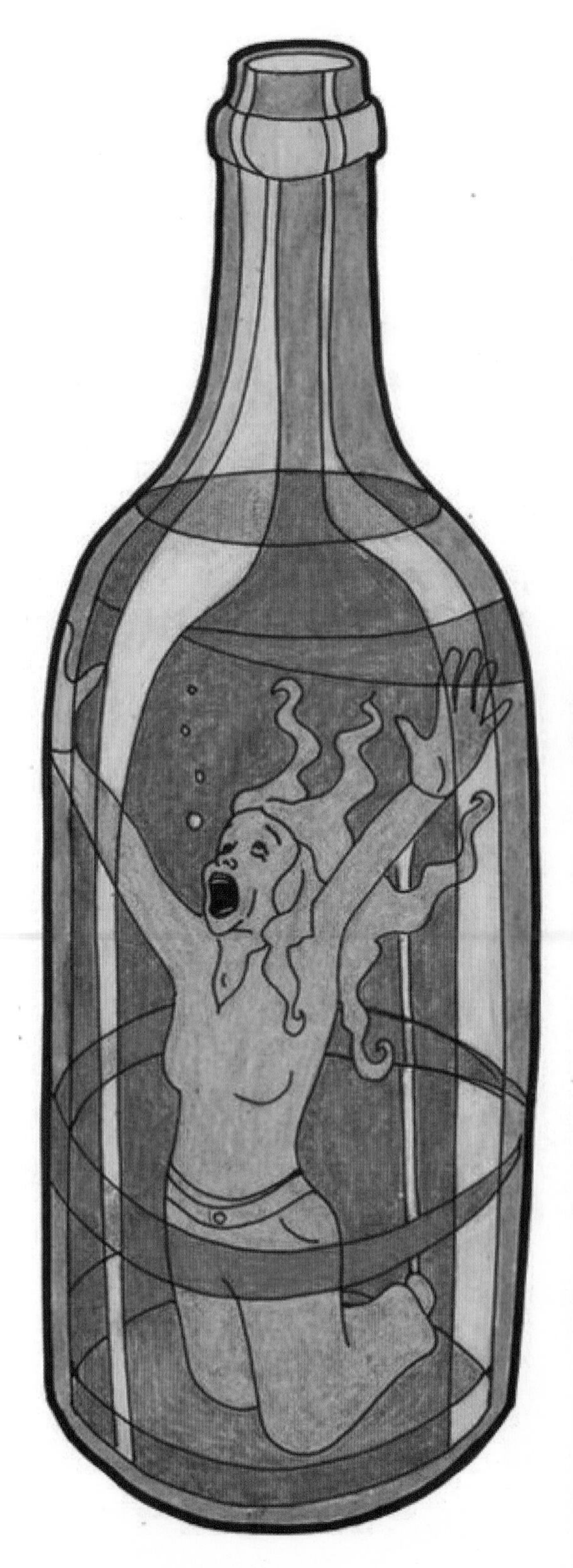

up my keys, dropping them, picking them up again, I moved towards the front door, opened it and began on my way – the walk to college. I knew there was a convenient off-licence nearby. By the time I actually reached the college, I'd consumed another half bottle of wine.

I slumped noisily into a seat and felt the warm, numbing feeling once again ebbing at my skull.

My pen scrawled across the paper. I knew my notes would be indecipherable later when I attempted to read them.

I could see and hear the lecturer at the front of the room. She paced slowly, back and forth, her clickety footsteps gradually annoying me, more and more.

My mind was fuzzy. It was 4.00 pm on a Friday afternoon: English Literature.

'MY ARSE,' I scribbled in the margin of a page, glancing sideways at my fellow student, Nicky. She smiled at the childish writing, the silly comment, but I could sense that the smile was rather forced.

I was growing tired, not listening with any real resolve to the lecturer's spiel. But I could just about tell that it was interspersed with the odd, supposedly witty comment from her, as I occasionally heard a laugh or two from my fellow students. I was oblivious to anything that was going on, in all honesty.

I lolloped back and forth in my seat, scrawling still, my mind a tangled mess. How the............. would I be able to make any sense of this rubbish later?

All I wanted, needed, was another drink.

Unprovoked

March 1992

My back ached as if my spine had morphed into a lead poker during the hours, endless hours I'd been sitting, or crouching, on the pavement of London's Chancery Lane. I did this most days, or at least every other day. I'd walk from Canning Town all the way to Chancery Lane to beg. I'd always be apprehensive when I arrived at my 'patch', but I'd gain confidence gradually when I'd made enough money to nip up the road to buy a couple of cans or a small bottle of brandy – then I could settle and concentrate on my daydreams of a better life.

My thoughts kept flicking around the welcome prospect of soon standing up and gathering together my rucksack and the rather elaborately painted sign, in vivid colours with stylized writing, saying loudly, but politely, 'PLEASE HELP, STUDENT, NO GRANT, NO LOAN, NO HOME'. (I had been a student but things had changed.) This was placed next to a manky old hat where a few coins lay. All of the pound coins and five pound notes had been quickly ferreted away in my various pockets and into my boots, out of sight.

My hand stretched to my coat pocket where I lovingly stroked the two twenties and the tenner given by three regulars I saw most days. A warmth spread through my body, seeping, comforting. Was it satisfaction though, or the effects of the three quarters of the bottle of cheap brandy I'd managed to obtain that morning? I couldn't decide.

Suddenly, I felt a smash against my head like an iron bar; catching me across my right cheekbone, pain splintering through my entire face with the speed of greased lightning. Immediately after this rock-hard blow to my face I realised I was being shoved forwards, downwards towards the kerb from behind. My left shoulder hit the ground. I heard a snapping, cracking sound.

I managed to twist my flailing, hurting body around and took the risk of peering up at my attacker. I screwed my eyes up as I turned to look round, feeling the expression of terror on my face. Terror mixed with a strange defiance, which surprised me.

I saw him. Dirty blond hair, stocky build, a grubby, chubby, sharp-eyed face, a grimacing snarly sneer... The thought, 'WHO THE HELL DO YOU THINK YOU ARE?' exploded in my mind just as another blow rained down onto my back, taking my breath away.

MY MONEY! I began scrabbling frantically through the pockets of my scraggy old coat...too late....my attacker was quick. His stubby fingers were rifling through my clothes, searching, poking, prodding. I managed to jerk my leg out, catching him with a satisfying crunch to his knee. He buckled slightly, flinching to one side, allowing me a moment's grace. My army boot managed to catch him again in the shin and I felt a fleeting flash of triumph as his cheeks reddened.

'YOU PIECE OF SHIT!' he growled down at me. Again, I fumbled for my stash of cash, feeling an alien triumph wash over me in an instant. He resumed his verbal attack.

'You little bitch! I've been watching you!' he sneered, his saggy face shaking and trembling with an incomprehensible rage against me.

'Give me that!' he grunted, once again grappling with my coat, one hand aiming a fierce punch to my throat. 'You filthy, little, begging, scrounging bitch,' he continued. I felt him reach the money and begin grabbing it from my pocket. Damn. No! 'You should be ashamed, you little shit!' He began shoving my money into his own pockets, dropping coins as he hurried. Occasionally he swiped at my face, yanked at my hair, pulling hard, grinning inanely at me. Eventually he took every penny I had. Six hours I'd been sitting there.

... he took every penny I had. Six hours I'd been sitting there.

I knew my begging was a risk I was taking. I understood how dangerous it was, but I hadn't expected THIS. That bastard had just come at me from bloody nowhere. I'd never even seen him before in my life.

'PEOPLE LIKE YOU SHOULD BE EXTINGUISHED!' he yelled. 'SCUM OF THE EARTH!' Even though he'd stolen every penny from me he still kept walloping me, as if he had some kind of pent up fury and he just HAD to get rid of it. On me!

'Begging slut,' he muttered, eventually turning away, brushing the front of his dirty jumper with his hands.

I winced at his words, feeling small and insignificant. So, as a beggar, I realised I was a target. I was a leech on society, a piece of scum.

The beginning of the end

August 1996

A sharp, agonising pain in my lower back caused my mind to become a messy blur.

Memories of 'when I was OK' combined with 'OH MY GOD, WHAT HAVE I DONE?' circled my befuddled brain like a hurtling ride at Alton Towers.

This pain, I knew, was serious. I knew I couldn't simply swallow a couple of paracetamol to get it to ease off.

Somehow I'd managed to end up at my parents' house and I was writhing around on the sofa whilst they looked on, debating what to do.

Suddenly, Mum seemed to have had enough of my groans of pain and announced she was calling the doctors' surgery. I made no argument; I knew I was in serious trouble.

I made no argument; I knew I was in serious trouble.

Equally as suddenly, I recognised the gnawing urge, want, need, I was harbouring for 'another drink', 'a big drink', 'a binge-drink'. I had to have a 'last one'.

Mum's voice informed me that I had to go to see a doctor 'IMMEDIATELY', and I began to protest that I would, but had to go to my flat first.

Being bundled into the car, all too soon I was in front of the doctor who wrote a letter for the attention of the hospital where I was to be admitted within the hour.

Again, my protesting arose, and I tried to establish an understanding that I MUST just pop into my flat for 'a few things' – LIE. I wanted that bottle of vodka I'd left on the coffee table – for God's sake, I'd only drunk half of it, damn it!

But, no! It wasn't to be, hospital it was for me, NOW. How would I survive without a drink, though?

GOD DAMMIT, my back felt as if it were exploding, something internally was very, very wrong. I could tell that, yet my frightened mind wouldn't allow me to dwell on that obvious fact.

My vision was blurred and I had an extreme pain in my back as I was wheeled into the hospital to a room all by myself. Ironically the TV was on, showing some intricate medical operation. Close-ups of blood and guts scared the living daylights out of me and the TV was quickly switched off.

I was semi-conscious when a syringe full of a thick, sticky-looking pink substance was injected into my arm. I was fixed up to a saline drip and told that I was 'Nil by mouth'. I insisted the door to my solitary confinement be left open. I felt so claustrophobic suddenly.

It must have been only fifteen minutes or so and I felt this huge, desperate urge for the loo – too late, a cascade of urine escaped me, a combination of embarrassment and relief washing over me as I looked in disbelief at the quantity of liquid which had exited my body. The floor was swimming – so that's why I was designated my own room.

The pain in my back began to ebb away. I had yet to find out that it was debatable whether my kidneys were failing; 'they' didn't know yet.

It was hopeless, my pathetic wishing that 'I hadn't got so bad', but right then I really wished I hadn't got so ill.

PLEASE give me a second chance, please.

I was delirious with a fever born of panic, yet I was exhausted and thankful to feel less pain.

A nurse cheerily entered my room, seemingly unperturbed by the sea of urine. She buzzed about, somehow manoeuvring me from the bed to a chair. She began stripping the bed, I began apologising wildly.

I dared to broach the subject of detox: 'Erm, d'you think I'll be starting a course of something to help stave off the withdrawal symptoms?' I asked, rather sheepishly, yet trembling inside.

'Oh, I don't know...' the nurse replied, 'You're not drinking anymore, so you'll be feeling better soon, I should think,' she said.

'Oh no,' I thought to myself. 'They don't get it about withdrawals and how they can cause fits or even heart failure.'

'I WILL need something like chlordiazepoxide or something,' I continued, but her expression was clueless. She may as well have been a truck driver who'd wandered into the hospital by mistake .

'PLEASE!' I heard my voice rising with panic, 'IT'S DANGEROUS TO JUST LET WITHDRAWALS HAPPEN – I'M REALLY SCARED.'

'Well,' she replied, 'you'll probably be seeing the doctor this afternoon...'

I felt a surge of anger at her rising in my throat. I knew, instinctively, what 'seeing the doctor this

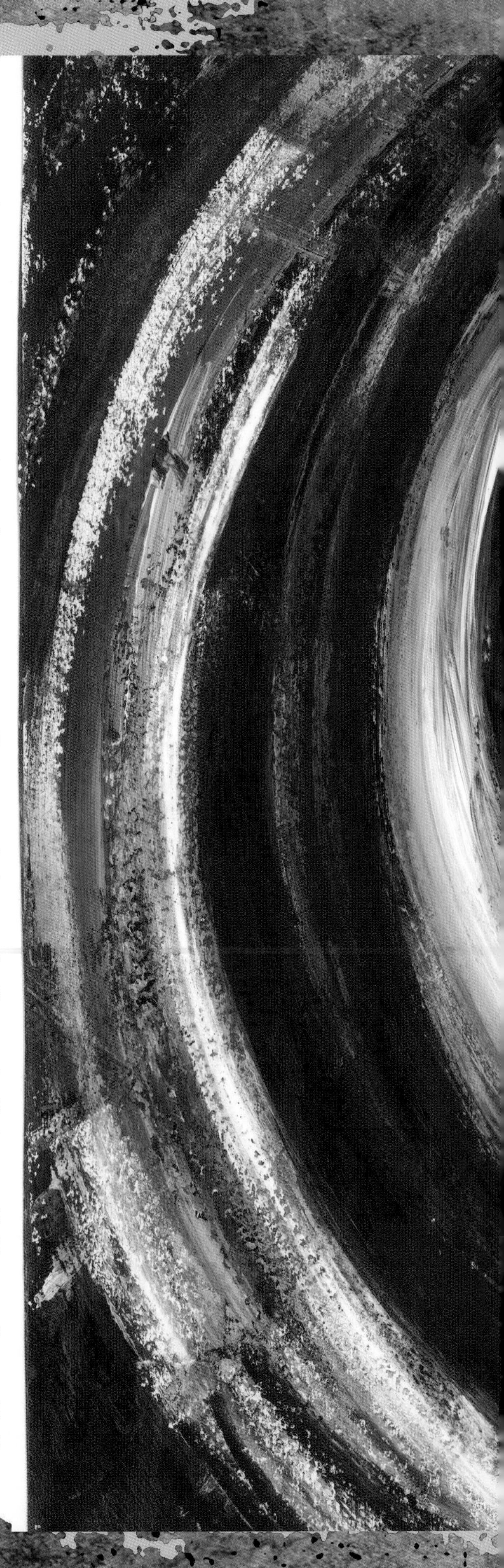

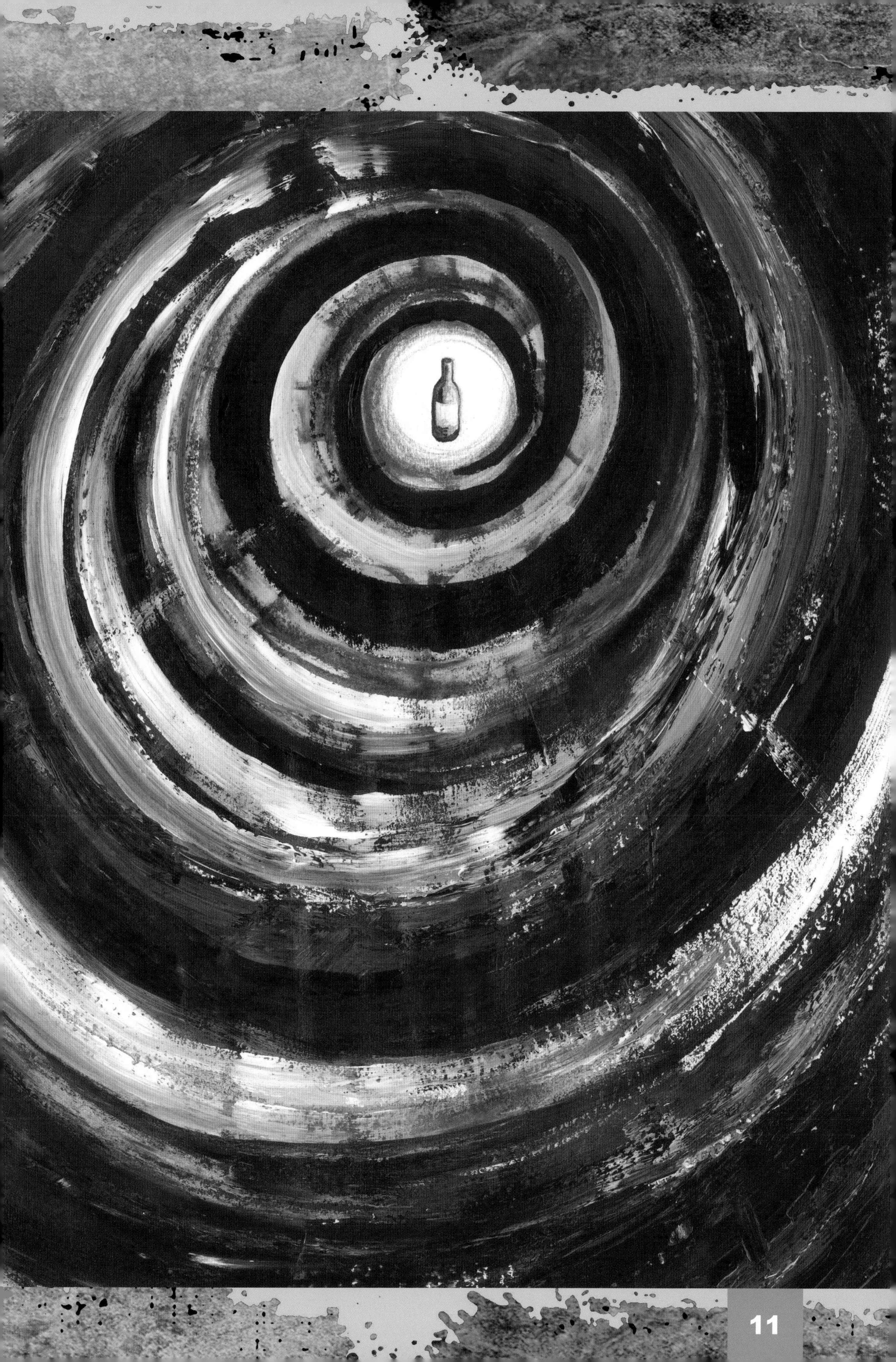

afternoon...' meant. It meant that I'd be discharged onto a general ward where a reluctant doctor would probably visit me the next morning or even later than that.

My mind was then made up.

I knew that I'd be better off just getting up and somehow making my way to see my own GP who was, of course, already up to speed on my situation. I hung on until word reached me that, yes, I was to be transported to a ward, then 'reassessed...' Hmm. I had already reassessed and my resolve was firm.

I knew that I'd be better off just getting up and somehow making my way to see my own GP...

I couldn't find my shoes! My cursing caused a nurse to appear at my door and, eventually, my shoes were found under my bed!

'I'm off...I have to go...self preservation...' I babbled.

'But...' she protested.

I dressed as best I could, fumbling, and unceremoniously pulled the drip tube from my hand, blood spurting out alarmingly as I did so. Ten minutes later I had discharged myself and was on my way to see my own GP who was expecting me. She consequently prescribed me medication to help my withdrawals.

I stopped drinking for roughly a week as I felt so unwell, but after that my drinking commenced yet again.

We were speeding, the small car juddering with exertion. Yet, somehow my friends seemed to understand the sheer desperation of the situation. No need for words. No conversation. Our rare 'day out' had taken on a shroud of darkness, of icy chill. My skin prickled with heartache as if my insides were working up to an alien-like osmosis ready to explode through my clammy, cold, outer shell.

My best friend, Lee, had automatically clasped my hand when I had answered my phone. He could tell by my distraught and disbelieving tone that something terrible had happened.

The telephone conversation had been quick yet life-changing. Shocking. Nightmarish.

My foot inadvertently connected with several empty beer cans and a half empty vodka bottle on the floor of the car, clanking my mind with a shooting pain over my left eye.

My sister, who'd called me, had said that Dad wasn't likely to 'have long left'.... My mind began to play tricks, what could that MEAN? It could mean that it was also likely that he DID have longer left, surely?

This was about the limit of my comprehension as alcohol, my first love, continued to befuddle my brain and meddle with my logic. I realised I'd been holding my breath. Lee still held my hand, his kind face scanning mine, pain etched into his pale skin.

The hospital came into view, grey, ominous, fear-inducing. It was filthy from the belching traffic fumes of the forever busy, traffic-laden road it was situated on. We stopped. The car was in the middle of the road and beeping and shouting began. My ears, however, were muffled and seemingly now immune to these everyday sounds. I looked at Lee's face as I flung open the back door of the car. He was ashen, grey as the hospital's dirty facade.

Running. Running.

I ran past crowds, dodged through traffic as car drivers cursed me.

Running. Running.

Through sliding doors which didn't slide fast enough.

Reception. Babbling my father's name and, 'Where is he?'

My heart. My heart.

Running to ICU.

I wished I had a drink with me.

Running.

My heart almost through my ribs.

Through the doors. Suddenly in a room.

Dad's face. My heart.

I noticed a smear of blood close to his lip. It was right next to the thick tube jammed into his mouth.

Respirator. My heart.

The sun shone through the grimy, fume-stained window of the white room as we made the decision to end my father's life.

My mother and sister were in the room with me. Mum was shaking. I didn't know what to do. I wanted to run and get alcohol as quickly as humanly possible to take this pain away. To kill it. Stifle it. Suffocate the hurting.

Dad looked.....like Dad.

Still breathing. His chest, up and down. Up and down.

My eyes wandered, vision cutting through the thick silence of the clinical intensive care room.

Big bucket container. Register.

Tube entering it. Register.

Blood. Register.

My heart.

My Dad. Bleeding.

Suddenly my heart leapt and I moved like a bullet shot towards him. Shook his shoulders. 'Wake up........'

Bleeding.

The sun shone through the grimy, fume-stained window of the white room as we made the decision to end my father's life. He had no gut anymore.

The small intestine. Gone. Infarction.

He'd gone into hospital to have a reversal operation of an ileostomy, so that he didn't have to wear ileostomy bags anymore. He was so happy when he got a date for the reversal operation.

Now his fate was decided.

Numb. Bleeding.

My heart.

Please let him open his eyes. Let me see the chocolate brown kindness again.

I desperately felt the pull of my alcoholism. It was calling me, calling me 'home'. I needed it. It didn't matter if I wanted it or not.

My heart. Bleeding.

I left it there. With Dad. My heart. With his.

I couldn't stay long. Alcohol called me with severe impatience. I had to obey.

I left my mother and my sister when they returned home.

Devastated. Numb. Bleeding.

I couldn't stay long. Alcohol called me with severe impatience. I had to obey. Alcoholism seemed to understand what I needed and its claws were ready to greet me, as ever.

Dad. Bleeding. Why did you leave me?

The sun shone on and I cursed it for doing so. Yet it didn't listen. It kept shining as I drank and drank.

Dad. Bleeding. DRINK. And the sun shone on.

Wake-up call

August 2004

The morning sun was much too bright for my tired, alcohol-fogged eyes. My bare feet were surrounded by empty bottles and a pint glass still full of white wine. The debris was the normal clutter to be found around me as I sat in my flat, alone.

My phone ringing broke the silence. My GP, Sally, wanted to see me immediately.

After guzzling the remainder of my wine, I managed somehow to reach the doctor's surgery. Sally's eyes betrayed her concern for me as I went into her room.

'Emma...' she began, looking at me in a different way than ever before. She had been my doctor for four years. She gestured me to sit down, but I couldn't still myself.

'Please, just tell me, what is it? Have they found something in the blood tests?'

Sally fixed me with her steady, blue gaze, 'Emma, all your stats are, well, all so wrong, so out of balance. To be honest your liver is starting to fail...you've got to do something NOW...you really have to...'

'What, am I ...have I got something, liver cancer or something, or?...' I began to jabber. I didn't want to contemplate something serious being wrong with me.

'You have considerable liver damage, yes. All of your results are pointing to your body just basically closing down.' Sally was speaking to me in a much more agitated fashion than her usual calm, serene way.

This rang alarm bells more loudly to me than anything else possibly could. Sally didn't get agitated. She was one of the calmest, most peaceful people I had ever met.

'PLEASE EMMA!' she ventured, 'Please don't let this happen to you.'

'But..' I interrupted.

'BUT ...WHAT? YOU ARE DYING, Emma.'

I couldn't quite believe how serious Sally was. I didn't WANT her to be that serious, dammit. What was she telling me? But I knew anyway. I knew. And I had tried for so long to block the reality out. Yet this was too sudden. God, I knew I had to decide. Could I decide?

I couldn't quite believe how serious Sally was.

Time stood still.

Stillness.

I could hear my own breathing. I could feel the thud of my own heart. My heart. I wanted it to continue beating, didn't I? I knew I wanted it to carry on thudding with life. I met Sally's eyes with my own. I sensed a tear begin to escape one of my eyes, to embark on its steady, hot roll down my cheek.

I felt regret for my lifestyle seeping from my every pore. Alcohol-soaked regret.

'I know...I will stop...now...' I spoke with an alien voice, trying to slow my heart.

'You must. Your body is telling you, "no more",' Sally replied.

'I'll need your help,' I said.

'It's a given...' she replied.

The decision was mine which path I took. Somehow it wasn't a difficult choice. I felt an inner calm, a resolve. I suppose I just wanted to live.

I felt my heartbeat slowing.

I knew I had to try.

I felt regret for my lifestyle seeping from my every pore. Alcohol-soaked regret.

Recovery

May 2013 ***Dedicated to Dr Sally Masheder***

My drinking life was an existence, it wasn't a life. It didn't resemble life as we know it, one iota. It was a chaotic, disturbing, disjointed state of being. Unpredictability became my unlikely companion as I continued my soulless quest to find solace in a bottle. The comfort and confidence that I had initially believed I'd discovered (like finding the Holy Grail or a lost text from Buddha) was quickly replaced with a physical craving for my daily intake of booze. It became a 'devil on my shoulder', one whispering in my ear that I needed alcohol in order to stay alive. I was a physical, mental and emotional wreck due to my copious drinking. I was allowing alcohol to destroy me and slowly kill me.

My drinking life was an existence, it wasn't a life.

The hurt and distress I caused to those close to me is, I know, irreparable damage. Yet, by staying sober, I know that I have begun to re-build bridges with family and close friends.

The contrast between then and now is the result, I believe, of a phenomenal spiritual change, along with the stark realisation that I had to alter my way of life entirely in order to stay alive. I was ready to embrace sobriety, although I was terrified of 'normal' life and not being numbed by the warm, yet vice-like, clutch of a drink. I still can't really comprehend how close to death I was on numerous occasions. Death or insanity were close by me for the years of my active alcoholism. I feel I walked, (or stumbled, crawled or crashed down flights of steps) with these two on each side of me. I was indeed, a crawling, disgusting mess.

The first step I had to take to stop drinking was to accept medication from my GP in order to prevent my withdrawal symptoms from becoming unbearable. The medication I was prescribed helped to minimize the delirium tremors (the shakes) and to calm me down as my body protested against not having alcohol on a daily basis. With perseverance, the violent shakes and tremors began to subside. My brain began to function again, focussing on more than the singular subject of alcohol and where the next load of it would come from. I began to realise that my drinking life was exhausted, spent. Over.

However, the most important thing for me and my recovery is the fellowship of Alcoholics Anonymous. I first attended an AA meeting when I was a teenager but I didn't fully appreciate its importance at that time. Now, the 12 step programme of AA enables me to meet and talk with other like-minded alcoholics about my life and experiences. To have a safe haven like AA where I can share my problems, feelings, and positive, happy things too, is an absolute Godsend.

Realising what I have lost through my drinking years is also a means to spur me on towards a positive future. I lost too many friends through my drinking. I also lost being involved with my family at important times, events and occasions. I say 'important times' but any time now with my family is important. When I was drinking I was very selfish. Alcohol came first, before anything or anyone. But my family were always there for me. They were there even when I thought they weren't.

I have had to distance myself from 'drinking friends'. Hard as this may be, I think it's vital for me to do this in order to stay strong in sobriety and to flourish in recovery.

I think that it is crucial that I try my best to fill my life with as much positivity and creativity as I possibly can. I realise how easy it is for me to 'slip' and lose my way in recovery. The path is often forked and I have to be careful which way I choose to go. During my drinking years I wrote copiously and then in recovery, I continued to write. My writing in sobriety became a kind of therapy for me and helped me to clarify my thoughts and feelings. It was an outlet for me to express myself. I also gained a Diploma in Counselling which I feel has also helped me to focus on my strengths.

Now, with clarity of mind, I know I have my life back. I know how I have damaged myself, much as I daren't think of this too often. I'm not as quick and fiery as I was before my onslaught from alcohol. My mind has suffered as well as my body. I have had to re-learn emotional responses which were damaged and twisted by alcohol.

I notice things now that I didn't used to pay attention to.

I feel privileged and fortunate beyond expression that I have, now, a good relationship with my mother, although I shall forever regret losing my father before he could get to know me again in my sobriety.

My life is no longer just an existence. I notice things now that I didn't used to pay attention to.

A kind word.

A breathtaking sunset.

The gift of true friendship.

The love and support of my mother.

The treasured memories of Dad.

Photographs which mean the world to me.

The re-forging of my relationship with my sister.

NO CHAOS.

I still get terrified! Some things throw me completely and I still feel greatly inadequate a lot of the time. But I am in a safe and wonderful place. The Esther Community has given me more hope, faith and nuggets of joy that I shall treasure always. My life is, for the most part, peaceful and productive now. I know that without drinking and the chaos and hurt it undoubtedly brings, things are probably going to be fairly fantastic.

2

hannah

The theme of Hannah's story is self-harming.

my story

I was born in Croydon in 1985 and when I was six I moved with my family to a little village called Rockbeare in Devon. I had a brilliant childhood there but when I was eleven my parents split up and I was told that my dad was not my real dad. I was devastated, angry and upset. He had been my role model, but from then on my relationship with him completely changed. I began to challenge his authority and I stopped feeling a part of the family.

We moved to Exeter, and I started to rebel. I hated school and I refused to go. I wanted so much to be popular but I had always been shy, and I felt unnoticed. I wanted to be noticed. I started smoking and drinking and experimenting with drugs. When I was thirteen I started self-harming. I used to burn myself with cigarettes and lighters because I thought I was a bad person and that I deserved pain. I would smash windows to harm myself and end up in hospital. This happened quite often during my teenage years.

When I was fifteen I left home. Life was up and down for me after that, as I was using drugs and drinking a lot. I fell out with my family because of my bad behaviour and the way I treated them. I started sofa surfing or sleeping on the streets. I was homeless for a few months and I moved into a hostel when I was sixteen. I managed to do two years at college, which I loved, but then my drinking got out of control. Because I had lost my family, I didn't care anymore and my drinking and drug-taking increased.

I attempted suicide on numerous occasions, usually as a cry for help. The most serious of these was when I jumped from a first floor window onto a pavement, breaking my back.

I moved into The Esther Community when I was eighteen and I have been there on and off ever since.

I aspire to be an author and a gym instructor.

The first cut

September 2001

I was sixteen. I had been at college all day and I was going out with my friends for a few drinks in the pub. I had had quite a few pints of beer but I was still with it and feeling very happy, having a laugh with my friends. We then decided to go to Tom's flat.

When we got there, one of the girls, who was by that stage really drunk, went into the kitchen, got a carving knife out of the drawer and said she was going to cut herself. At first I tried to talk her out of it. But then, something happened in my head, and I grabbed the knife out of her hand and slashed at my arm really hard, four times. I didn't feel any pain. I sank to the floor. There was blood everywhere. I was screaming and crying. She grabbed the knife from me and started trying to comfort me. Then all my other friends, hearing the commotion, came rushing into the kitchen and surrounded me, trying to calm me down, while Tom rang for an ambulance. I was hysterical but I was also the centre of attention. Why had I grabbed the knife off her? I didn't really want to hurt myself. Was it because I didn't want her to be the centre of attention? I wanted to be the centre of attention and I copied her idea. I had always been so desperate to be noticed and now, by cutting myself in this extreme way, I had achieved just that.

I had always been so desperate to be noticed and now, by cutting myself in this extreme way, I had achieved just that.

In the hospital my whole family came to see me and I loved the attention. I was laughing and joking with them and the nurses. This was what I wanted my life to be like. When I left hospital and went home my family continued to make a fuss of me. They cooked me my favourite meal – Mexican fajitas, and hired DVDs they knew I would like. It was so nice, but it so rarely happened.

But after a while the attention wore off, and my mind became full of different emotions. I felt embarrassed, guilty and then extremely depressed. I couldn't believe I had done something so drastic just to feel noticed and get attention. I had been so selfish and I was now in quite a lot of pain as I had cut the tendons in my arm and had had to have an operation.

I hid away in my attic bedroom. I sat on my wooden bed, drinking lager and listening to music, not really knowing what to do with myself. I felt so depressed and didn't want to see anyone. My life went back to normal but I was still lonely and I carried on drinking.

That was the first time that I cut myself, but for the same reasons I did it quite a few more times after that.

Escape

October 2010

I woke up, still feeling slightly drunk and spaced out from the medication I had taken the night before. But nothing had changed. I still felt trapped and depressed. Everything had gone downhill since I'd moved back in with my mum four months before and I couldn't believe where my life was now. It was so different from where I was six months ago and all I could think was, 'I really want my life back. I want to be back at The Esther Community, clean from drugs and keeping fit and healthy.' But I had no one to talk to, no friends and no help. I was alone in a flat with my mum – day in, day out. Now, all I wanted was to be as far from reality as possible. So I did the only thing I knew how, which was to take some more valium and go and watch some TV in the front room.

I was alone in a flat with my mum – day in, day out. Now, all I wanted was to be as far from reality as possible.

As I sat there, all I could think about was hurting myself and then I thought, 'I want to jump out the window. I want to jump out the window.' I walked to the window and opened it. I looked out and I thought, 'Oh my God, stop being stupid.' I then went back to the sofa and continued watching the TV. The medication I had taken started to make me feel a lot further from reality.

My mum then walked into the front room and said, 'All you do is get up late and sit in front of the TV. You never do anything!' I couldn't believe what she was saying. Since I'd moved in all I had done was clean, cook and do everything for her. I felt like a slave. I shouted back at her which caused a major argument. We were both swearing at each other and then she hit me.

I pushed her away and said, 'Right, I'm going to jump out the window.'

'Don't be so stupid,' she said.

But as I got closer to the window all I could think was, 'I need to escape. I need to get out of this situation.' I then climbed onto the window sill and jumped. It felt really surreal, like I was in a dream, only this was my reality. And then, suddenly, it was over. As I lay on the concrete, I tried to move, but couldn't, and I tried to speak, but no words would escape my lips.

Mum shouted, 'Stay there, I'm going to call an ambulance.'

While I lay there waiting I didn't feel any pain. After that, I don't remember much. The ambulance came and I remember they had to cut my hoodie off and I didn't want them to. After that my mind was blank. When I woke up and looked around me, I was in hospital and I couldn't move. The pain was immense, but all I could think was, 'Yes, I have escaped.'

I broke my back, heel, ankle and wrist. I was in hospital for six weeks and the pain I felt was indescribable. My mother came to visit me but it was awkward. I felt numb. She asked me if I regretted what I I'd done but I said, 'No.' My head was all over the place. I was getting attention, which I loved, so in some ways I didn't regret it and I had, after all, managed to get out of living in my mother's flat. But if I hadn't been using so many drugs, I don't think I would have done something quite so drastic.

When I left hospital I was put into a bedsit with a wheelchair. I really hated not being able to walk and being stuck indoors all day. I still felt very lonely as I didn't have many visitors and it took me at least six months to walk again. When I did finally start walking it felt great, although I couldn't walk very far at first, because of the pain. Now, nearly three years later, my walking has really improved.

My relationship with my mother went back to how it was, but we never really talked about what had happened. We have always had big arguments and fights and we normally end up laughing about it in the end. It is a real love-hate kind of relationship, and even though I know I cannot live with her, I do love her because, whatever happens, she is always there for me.

I decided to try the public toilets; not the most luxurious of places for a girl and her diamonds.

I was bored. I had some money and decided to treat myself to a few stones of crack. I felt really excited at the thought of having another pipe. I rang my dealer and asked where we should meet. It was always somewhere miles away, but my mind was made up. There was no going back.

I got there and, as I was walking to meet him, I felt impatient and greedy for the buzz. I was almost running to get to the meeting place. All I could think about was the first pipe, the taste. I was salivating at the thought. I wanted it now. I wanted it badly. It was almost as if I was buzzing already. I got to the place and rang him. He said he'd be there in five minutes. All I could think was, bollocks, he was never on time, but I would wait. I wouldn't have left for anything. My thoughts kept drifting to the first pipe I would soon be enjoying. The first pipe is always the best. I felt like a little kid at Christmas waiting to unwrap that first present. Then I saw him strolling towards me and my face lit up. I jogged up to him and handed him the money. He handed me the stones. As soon as they were in my hand they felt like diamonds, precious diamonds, and all for me.

I made my way back to town, walking with speed. I had to find somewhere to go. I decided to try the public toilets; not the most luxurious of places for a girl and her diamonds. I could feel the excitement bubbling up inside me. I couldn't believe

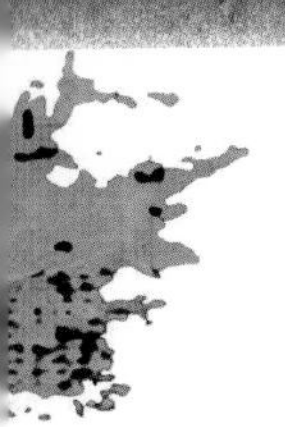

these rocks could make me feel so euphoric. I wanted this feeling to last forever. But it never does.

I finished the last stone and all I could think was, 'I want more, I want more,' but I had no more money. I wondered why I'd spent all my money on an amazing buzz that had lasted for such a short time and now I was thinking of ridiculous ways of getting more money.

I made my way back to The Esther Community, still on a bit of a high, but £80 lighter. I decided to watch a bit of TV and chill out, but I felt slightly on edge and restless, and then I started to feel extremely low with different questions beginning to rush through my head. Why had I spent all my money? What was I going to live off for the next two weeks? Why had I been such an idiot? Why did I keep making the same mistakes over and over again? I now felt really depressed and annoyed with myself. I really needed someone to talk to. My mum seemed like the perfect person, but I couldn't get hold of her. Now I was feeling worse. I wanted these feelings to go but the questions and thoughts kept flooding my head. They wouldn't stop and they kept on coming. It was overwhelming.

I decided to go to my room to try and clear my head and also to try and contact my mum again, but without any luck. I wanted this to end. I could feel tears welling up and then something inside me took over. I grabbed some tablet boxes and started popping out as many pills as I could. I ate them as if they were a packet of sweets. Just as I had swallowed the last pill my phone rang. It was my mum. Why now? Why not fifteen minutes earlier? I answered and told her what I'd done and begged her not to tell the staff or ring an ambulance. I said I was going to go straight to bed and sleep it off.

Just as I had swallowed the last pill my phone rang. It was my mum. Why now? Why not fifteen minutes earlier?

When I put the phone down I did feel a lot better but it was too late to undo what I had done. My mum didn't ring the staff, she phoned one of my friends instead and the next thing I knew there was a knock at my door. It was two of my friends and they saw all the tablet wrappers and knew something wasn't right. I tried to convince them that everything was OK, I just wanted to get into bed and go to sleep. But it was not to be. Two minutes later the staff were at my door and the next thing I knew I was in an ambulance and on my way to hospital. Luckily for me, I was OK and I was discharged the next day.

When I came back to The Esther Community I felt stupid but still very depressed. Why did I keep doing this, making the same mistakes over and over again? I didn't know.

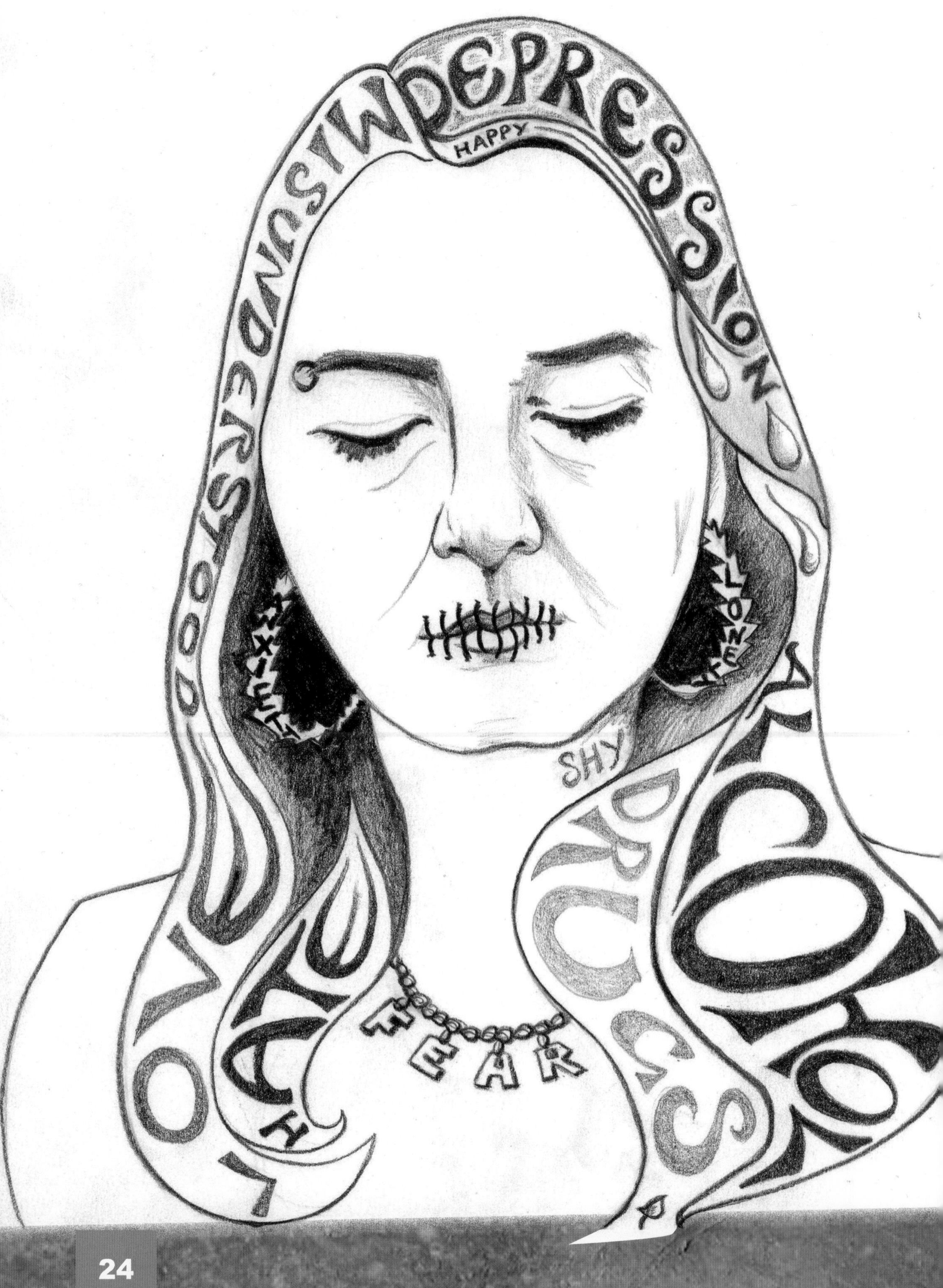
DEPRESSION
HAPPY
MISUNDERSTOOD
SHY
FEAR
DRUGS

New beginnings

May 2013

I stopped self-harming when I was twenty-one. Through the help that I have received, I realised that I was not a bad person and I could be myself. I now finally feel comfortable with who I am. I also feel more able to deal with my emotions and to cope in stressful situations. There was an occasion recently when I went through a difficult time. In the past I would have attempted to take my life as a way out from that situation, but this time I somehow found it within myself to get through it, and come out the other end, still in one piece. I felt proud of myself.

I have successfully come off heroin and amphetamines. I decided to come off heroin because I didn't want to be that person any more. For three years, on and off, my life just revolved around scoring and getting high. I didn't do anything else. I had a chance to detox and be titrated in a hospital. I took that chance and it worked. I have not used heroin again. Seeing how ill other people can be on heroin and some of the things they have to do to get a fix really stops me from going back on it. Some of my best friends are addicted and I have seen how badly it changes them and destroys them. I have now been clean for two years. I feel I have got my personality back and my sense of humour. I now know there is more to life than just being high. There are times now when I feel high from life, and that feels so much better than taking any drug.

The main thing that I think has helped me to overcome my problems is talking to people and getting my thoughts and feelings out.

My drinking is now also under control. I detoxed and didn't drink for four years. I am now able to have a social drink without the worry of it escalating. I know when to stop.

The main thing that I think has helped me to overcome my problems is talking to people and getting my thoughts and feelings out. Talking about things helps me sort them out in my head. I talk to the staff at The Esther Community, drug workers and close friends. They all help me in different ways. I think it is far better to ask for help rather than keep it all inside and then let it come out in all the wrong ways.

I don't always find it easy to express myself, but I have found that writing about the events of my past and the things I have done helps me to piece things together and to understand myself and my behaviour.

I have now made up with my family. I still feel very guilty about the way I treated them but I am gaining their trust. Although I don't see them often, I am glad they are back in my life and I hope to see them a lot more often.

In a way I'm glad I've gone through what I've gone through, as I know I am now a stronger person. I also know there are a lot of other people like me and I am not alone. I'm now, finally, feeling much more positive about my future.

anna

The theme of Anna's story is domestic violence.

3

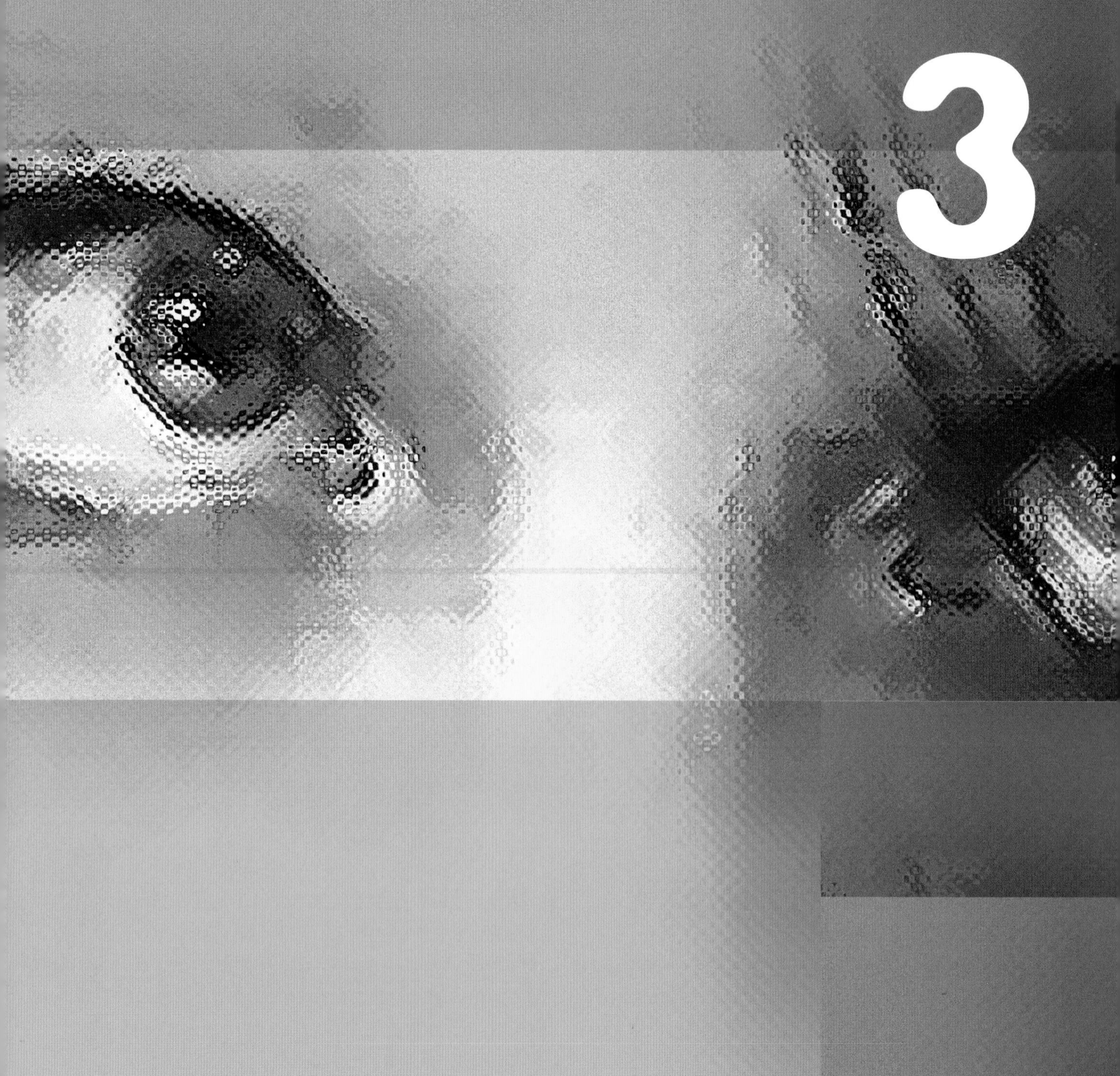

my story

I was raised in Nottingham. I was a rebellious teenager and got into drugs and alcohol at a young age. I moved into the YMCA and lived there for a couple of years. It was there that I met my husband. We married very quickly and had three children. We stayed together for ten years and although he was a good man it just never seemed enough for me and we split up. I thought at the time it was what I wanted but I didn't cope very well and after that my drinking and drug habits got worse.

And then, I met Rob. I adored him, but even from the start the relationship was unhealthy. My drug intake increased, resulting in a crack cocaine habit, and I started drinking every day. My children ended up living with my parents and I was stuck in a violent relationship that just got worse and worse. Before I knew it I was isolated from my friends and family and under the control of an abuser. I had two more children but because of my drug and alcohol problems, they too went to live with family members.

It took me years to realise what was happening to me. I finally found the strength to leave Rob after ten years of abuse. I do believe that if I hadn't left when I did I would have been seriously injured or dead within a few years.

Now I am rebuilding my life and I would like to help other women who have suffered domestic violence and abuse.

I aspire to be an author.

Turning point

September 2006

I lay on the bed in the side room. Although the door was shut, I could still hear the babies crying and the sounds of the other mothers wheeling their cots to the changing room and feeding room to tend to their little ones. I looked up to the drip in my arm which contained fluids and antibiotics that were being pumped into me. My stomach hurt from the c-section that I had had the day before.

My body was aching but it wasn't as bad as the ache that I felt deep inside my heart. Every time I heard one of the other babies cry, I wanted my baby, my little girl. I wanted to hold her, to feed her, to change her. I hadn't even got to see her yet. I knew she was OK and was doing well. She had not been born dependent on the drug that I was stupidly addicted to. My mum was with her and she was healthy. She would be allowed to go home with my mum and dad and be with her brothers and sisters. It was a huge relief. Our little girl would not be going into care, but a part of me hated it too, hated the fact she was not with me. I sobbed into my pillow, my nighty becoming wet from my milk. I wanted to nurse my baby so much.

My little girl, my perfect little girl, a full head of hair, beautiful and innocent. How could I have been so stupid to have put her in any danger?

The door opened. It was time. Finally I would get to hold her. And there she was: my little girl, my perfect little girl, a full head of hair, beautiful and innocent. How could I have been so stupid to have put her in any danger? It was so emotional. My mum cried. I cried. I didn't get to hold her for long. Then my mum took her home and even though I knew she was safe and would want for nothing, it was at that moment that my heart broke. I had never felt so much pain before. Every beating, every black eye, bruise or cut was nothing compared to the pain of this.

I don't know how long I lay there and cried before Rob came in. Neither of us said a word. He just walked in and held me. We both sobbed as we held each other. He lay down on the bed next to me and held me as we cried. He stroked my hair and tried to comfort me, telling me softly that everything would be ok, that together we would get things sorted. I felt so close to him. He was the only one who understood how I felt. I drifted off in his arms.

I got stronger as the days went by. It wasn't long before I was allowed to go home. Rob was brilliant; he was my rock. When we got home he had made a bed up for me in the living room so that he could be with me all the time. He did everything for me: cooked, cleaned, helped me bathe and dress my wound. We would lie there and talk about how things were going to be different. We were going to give up the drugs and prove to everyone that we could be the perfect family. When Rob was loving and caring he was everything I wanted – kind, considerate and protective. I would completely fall for his charm and believe his lies. He had a way of making me feel that I couldn't live without him. But he had isolated me from other people so much that he was all I had left and all I wanted and all I thought I needed. I was so utterly blinded I really believed him when he promised he would change. But it didn't last for long.

It was roughly two weeks after I had been home and I felt restless. I was able to move around really well and we had been so good. No drugs. But one day we decided to have a drink. It was late afternoon and we decided to venture out and take a trip over to Rob's mum's place. We grabbed some more beer and we caught a bus.

The bus journey over to his mum's took about half an hour. We both carried on knocking down the beers. Rob was beginning to get tense and started asking me questions. Questions like, 'You would never cheat on me would you?'

And then he said it: 'The baby is mine, isn't she?'

I couldn't believe it. I was instantly hurt, angry and upset. 'How could you even think that?'

'It goes through my head sometimes,' he said.

I grabbed his face in my hands and looked him straight in the eyes. 'Rob, I would never cheat on you. I love you with all my heart. She is yours.'

'OK,' he said.

Sometimes he would get paranoid and sometimes he would need reassurance but for him to even ask - that really upset me. I guess the drink made the situation more tense but for the rest of the bus journey the atmosphere between us got colder.

'Why the fuck have you got so stroppy? Have I hit a nerve?' he said.

I just shot him a look. I did not want to have a row with him on the bus in front of people. It was getting dark outside and our stop was coming up.

I could instantly see his eyes had changed. He wanted a row.

'I must have hit a nerve you whore. You're not denying it,' he hissed at me as he stood up and went to the front of the bus.

My cheeks were flushed red with embarrassment and anger. How could he even think anything like that? The bus stopped and we got off. He marched on ahead of me. I didn't want this. I didn't want a row. So I walked fast to catch up with him, pleading with him, stupidly trying to reassure him. We arrived at the entrance to the park which was a shortcut to his mum's. He was still slightly ahead of me. I could hear him muttering but couldn't hear what he was saying.

'Oh, for fuck's sake! If you have something to say, just say it,' I said.

He turned round and came marching towards me. As he did, I could instantly see his eyes had changed. He wanted a row.

'Ok you slag. Who's the fuck is she, because

she ain't mine? I can see it in your face.'

'Oh fuck off. She is yours and you know it. Why are you doing this?'

'Because you are a no-good, cheating slag. She's not mine is she?'

And then I did the most stupid thing ever. Because of how absurd his accusations were and because I knew one hundred percent that she was his child, I rolled my eyes and said, 'Yeah right, she's not yours. I've been leading you on all this time. Whatever.'

His brain did not compute the sarcasm in my voice. In his head it was an admission. And there it was. Bang! His fist hit me straight in the mouth. I staggered back and before I even had the chance to register the punch he had one hand grabbing my hair and the other around my throat.

'You dirty slag. I'm gonna kill you.'

He spat in my face and pushed me down onto the ground. My eyes were bulging, I couldn't get a breath. I tried to pull his hand off my throat but he was too strong. He was pushing down on my throat and I could feel myself go light headed. I was gasping for air, my heart was pounding. I was kicking, pleading with him through my eyes.

His phone rang. He let go of my throat and I sat there gasping. It was his mum.

He screamed at her, 'Mum, I swear I'm gonna kill her. This dirty whore has been lying to me. I'm on my way with her. She can tell you about it, the bitch.'

He hung up and then turned on me, grabbing my hair and kicking me. It had only been a couple of weeks since my c-section and I curled up trying to protect the area from the kicks. I still had my stitches in. He started to drag me by the hair. I could feel my thigh grazing on the path as he dragged me, still kicking me and screaming at me to get up.

'GET UP YOU BITCH OR I SWEAR I'LL FUCKING KILL YOU.'

I don't know how I managed to get up but I did. I remember swaying and him grabbing me again and marching me through the park. He grabbed my head in his hands and screamed obscenities into my face and then he head-butted me. I must have blacked out because when I came to I was in the graveyard that ran along the path to his mum's. To get there we would have had to go across the main road and down another path, and I have no memory of how we got there. I was lying across a grave, my head against the stone edging. The pain in my shoulder was excruciating. I realised he was biting me.

'Please stop,' I begged.

'STOP? Fucking stop? I ain't even started, you slag.'

His face was pressed against mine, his teeth gritted. He was talking to me in what could only be described as a snarl.

'I'm gonna kill you tonight, you whore. I'm gonna rape you and kill you. You will never see your kids again.'

That's when I felt it against my neck, the cold steel blade of the Stanley knife. I froze.

I looked into his eyes. I really thought he would kill me. I thought I was going to die. And then, all I could think about were my babies, my beautiful children. The thought of never being able to hold them, talk to them, tell them that I loved them was too much. I began to cry.

'Please Rob. Just let me go. Please. If I go you will never hear from me again. Please, please, please,' I begged, sobbed and pleaded with him.

'If I let you go you will tell the police you grassing scum.'

'I won't. I'll just go home,' I said.

He lowered the knife.

'Get up,' he said, 'we're going to my mum's.'

I got up and began to stagger in the direction of his mum's, begging him to let me go. He marched beside me, every now and then giving me a slap round my head. We carried on like this for the rest of the journey which took about ten minutes. We got to his mum's and she must have heard her gate open as she opened the door to greet us. The smile vanished from her face when she saw my beaten, swollen face. He pushed past her and went in. She grabbed me.

'What happened?' she said.

'Please. I just want to go home,' I sobbed.

He was shouting from inside the house, shouting for his mum to bring me in. I looked at her and begged her to let me go. A friend of mine lived around the corner. I wanted to get there. I would be safe there.

'Go, quick,' she said.

I stumbled to the gate and out into the road. I thought I was going to be OK. It was over, wasn't it? I heard my name being called and I turned round just in time to see him drop kick me to the head. Blood sprayed out as I fell to the ground. One of my eyes was already closed and swollen. My lips were split and I could feel part of my mouth hanging down, split from the rest.

Why was he doing this?

Then he was on top of me, banging my head on the road. There were people around now. A few of them tried pulling him off me but he was like a crazed animal and kept coming back, hitting, kicking, biting. I kept blacking out. I remember seeing the flashing blue lights and people dragging him off me. I don't know how I got up but I managed it and I got to my friend's door. I banged on it and fell against it. She did not recognise me.

Time went by in a daze. The ambulance came. They put me in one of their seats and they wheeled me out. I looked up the street and I could see the police had Rob in restraints. He was handcuffed and they had strapped his legs together. He had at least three officers sitting on him. It was stupid but I wanted to protect him. I was worried they would hurt him. Crazy, I know.

There wasn't a part of my body that didn't have a cut or a bruise. They told me at the hospital I was lucky to be alive. My lip was split wide open, my eye socket fractured and cut open. They said that I was lucky

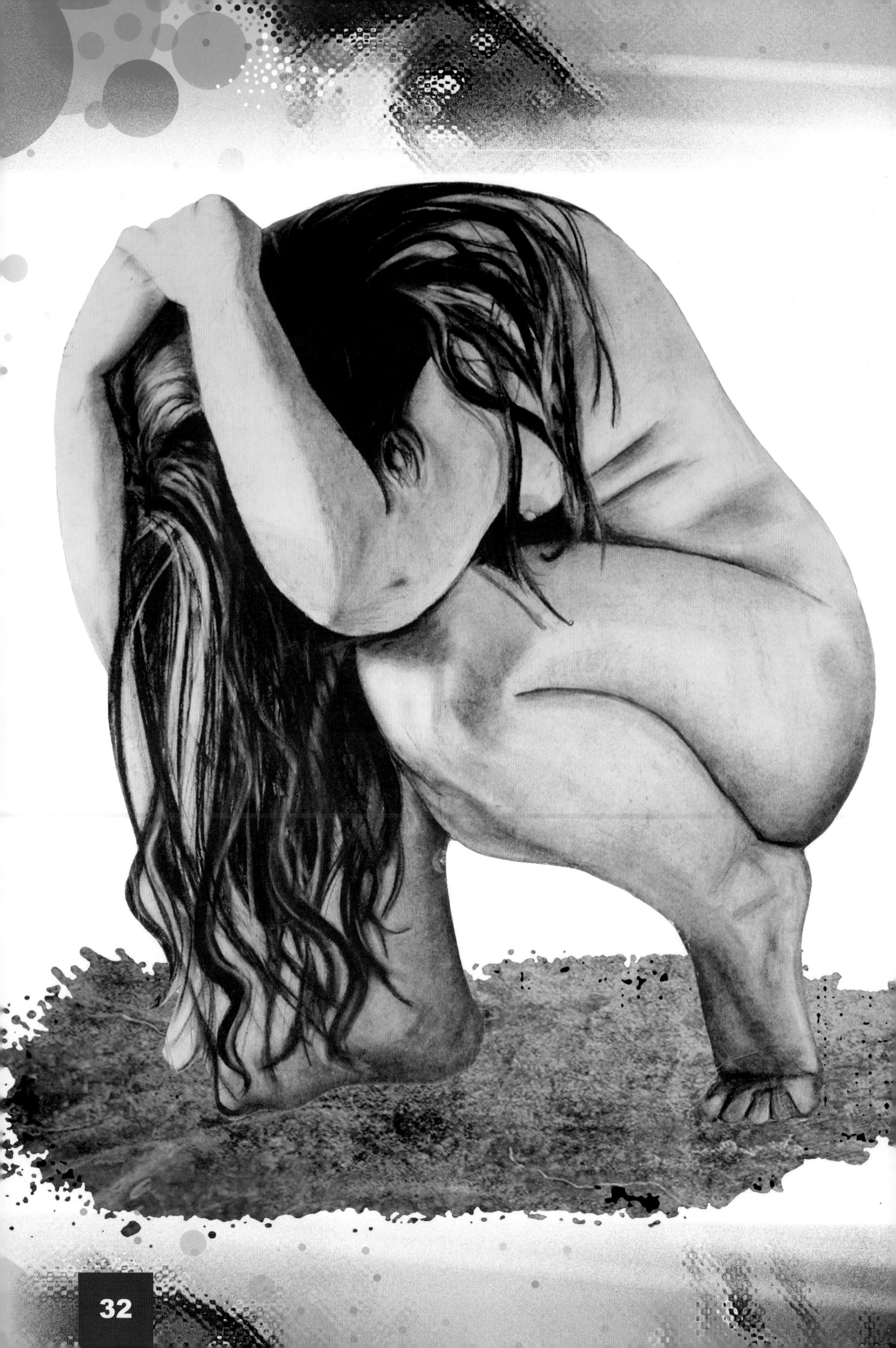

that the kicks to my stomach did not reopen my c-section. If that had happened I would have bled to death in seven minutes.

I later found out that the twenty minutes it should have taken to get from the bus stop to his mum's took over three hours. What had happened? Where had the time gone? I was scared to remember.

I wear the scars from that night and I still to this day have nightmares about it. But it didn't stop me going back. The phone calls started. At first I ignored them but after a few days I started to miss him. I think it was because the attack had come from nowhere and I wanted to hear from him. Why had he done this to me? I started to speak to him on the phone, listening to him apologising, pleading with me, begging me. His crying always pulled my heart strings. But he didn't do it much. He was too hard for that. But there he was, crying, promising that he would change, promising that he would get help. I really believed him and I went back after two weeks. Before I went back he had started to put things in place. He went to the doctor's and probation and told them he needed help. I went with him on a few occasions. I really hoped that this time it would work. After all, it couldn't get any worse. Could it...?

It was nearly the same ritual every morning. He would be cursing and I would be running round trying to get all the bits he needed together whilst trying to be as unnoticeable as possible.

I awoke to him shouting. I lay there and thought, 'Here we go, just another day and by the sound of it he is in one of those moods. Just another day.'

I had begun wondering just lately, wondering why I bothered. Would today be the day? The 'normal' day that in my heart I truly desired. The day that the light finally switched on in his head and at last he realised that I was not his enemy. I was the one person that truly loved him.

The sound of banging and crashing and him saying, 'Where the fuck are they?' awoke me from my thoughts.

With a sigh I got out of bed, put my dressing gown on and called out, 'Hey, what's wrong?'

'I can't find my fucking boots,' was his reply. I rolled my eyes as I walked into the hallway and went to the spot under the stairs where his boots were put last night. Still listening to the cursing and obscenities that came from his mouth, I picked up his boots and called to him that I had found them. I knew full well that his mood was not about his boots at all and it was just him being him. I also knew that I had to tread carefully and not give him any excuse to take his mood out on me.

I put his boots down in front of his chair and went to the kitchen to make his coffee and grab his lunch. I had already prepared it last night and put it in a bag ready for him to take to work. It was nearly the same ritual every morning. He would be cursing and I would be running round trying to get all the bits he needed together whilst trying to be as unnoticeable as possible.

'What are your plans for today?' he asked.

'Oh, not much,' I replied. 'Just the usual housework, shopping, plus I have a doctor's appointment today.'

He came towards me, put his fingers through my hair and gripped really hard, pulling my head back, his face close to mine and through gritted teeth he said, 'I think maybe you should cancel your appointment. You don't want them to see what a clumsy bitch you are, now do you?' I winced under his grip, knowing full well that he meant that he did not want the doctor to see the bruises that had appeared on my stomach and chest from last night's angry fit.

'OK, OK,' I pleaded, 'I'll ring them and tell them I can't make it. I'll ask them for a prescription.'

'That's a good girl,' he said and kissed me. 'Where's my bag?'

'I'll just get it babe,' I said, relieved to be out of his grip. He put his boots on and I grabbed everything he needed. With a kiss he was out of the door.

Three weeks. That was all it had been since I had decided to give him another go and try again. Three weeks was all I needed to realise that he was never going to change. I had spent the last four months away from him. Four months of beginning to be me again after ten years. Four months being able to wake up in the morning without the worry of upsetting him. Four months without living in fear and dread. But, and I know this sounds crazy, four months of missing being wrapped in his arms in bed at night, missing his protectiveness. He was my drug and wow had he got me addicted!

I made myself a cup of tea and watched Jeremy Kyle on telly. My 'me time', I chuckled to myself. Afterwards, I rang the doctor and arranged to pick up the prescription. Then I did the housework and all the time my mind was in torment, wondering what Rob's mood would be like on his return. Did I want this anymore? Was I strong enough? The day went on as normal. I managed to relax a bit until it got closer to the time when he came home.

The car pulled up in the driveway. I watched through the window as Rob's friend Kevin got out of the car and I opened the door. Rob was getting into the driver's seat with his can of Stella. I could see that he was already drunk.

'Get in the car,' Kevin said. Without hesitation I grabbed my jacket. Only a few seconds had passed and already Rob was honking the horn. Kevin and I shared a nervous glance. Although we never said anything, we both understood, we both went through the same thing every day. Kevin was just as abused as me. He suffered just as much as me, day in, day out.

I grabbed my keys, my phone and anything else I thought we might need and I shut the door behind me. When I got in the car I could smell the drink and I could see how drunk he was.

'Alright babe?' he grinned at me as he lent in to kiss me. On the outside he seemed quite cheery but I knew it would only be the slightest thing that would kick him off. As we drove, they recounted their day. Of course there had been some drama. He was bragging about how he had told someone at work about himself. Just the usual.

I was in my own little world as they laughed and joked about their day. I felt bored, bored of the same trivial drivel that came from his mouth. Did I really want this anymore? Why was I still here? I deserved more. Didn't I? I was in my own world and did not notice the beep on my phone to let me know that I had a message.

'Who's that?' he asked.

'I don't know,' I said as I nervously looked at my phone. It was from my friend David. The text was innocent. All it said was, 'Hey how's things?' But just an innocent text like that was enough.

David and I had been friends for years, since back in the days when I was a carefree teenager. There had been a group of us who had all lived together in the same hostel. We had all kept in contact with each other over the years and been to each other's weddings. But, gradually, contact with any of them had become less and less because of my relationship with Rob. Friends, family and any sort of contact with anyone other than him would fuel his paranoia and would wind him up. I had come to realise over those four months just how isolated I had become. And why? Just to keep the peace? I had realised a lot over those four, Rob-free months. I had realised just how much of a prisoner I had become. It had become an automatic reaction to avoid anyone or anything that would wind him up and annoy him: a kind of defence mechanism. But in those four months I had started to renew some of my old friendships again. And there it was: an innocent text from an old friend that triggered the events of the start of my new life.

I had come to realise over those four months just how isolated I had become.

He grabbed my phone. I was already scared and curled against the side of the car door, waiting, already in a defensive position; waiting for what I knew was coming. It had happened so many times before although this time it felt different somehow. I felt different. I had realised a long time ago that it did not matter what I said to him or how much I denied it.

'YOU DIRTY CHEATING WHORE,' were the words that came from his mouth as he punched me in the side of the head, the phone still in his clenched fist. He stopped the car so he could hit me more easily. He continued to hit me as he reached over and opened the car door, pushing me almost out of it, but at the last minute grabbing my hair, and pulling me back. He started the car again and began to drive with me half-hanging out of the door, but the door kept swinging back and hitting me in the head. He stopped the car again and somehow got into a position so he could kick me with both feet. He started screaming at Kevin, 'GET THIS SLAG OUT OF MY CAR.' Without hesitation, Kevin jumped out and tried to pull me out. But it was no use. The door would not open because of the grass verge in the way. Realising this, Rob moved the car forward, with Kevin running to keep up, until there was enough room for the door to open and me to be chucked out. I landed hard on the side of the road. Kevin jumped back into the car and they drove off.

I lay there, at the side of the road, curled up, blood and tears running down my face, wincing from the pain on my grazed palms. It was getting dark and my body hurt. It took all my strength to get up. I was sobbing but relieved it was over. I began to walk and then I saw a car approaching. But because of the tears in my eyes and the glare of the lights I could not make out what car it was until it was practically on top of me. The fear and panic I felt when I saw it was him was immense.

I began to run. He drove beside me, demanding that I get into the car. Then his demands turned into pleading, and it's crazy, but I began to soften towards him. No, not soften, weaken. He stopped the car and got out, and began jogging beside me, pleading with me to let him take me home, telling me how sorry he was, how wrong he was to have hit me. There was no aggression left in his voice and like a fool I stopped walking. I just stood there and sobbed, my head hung low, my arms limp by my side. I was not thinking, my mind was blank as I let myself be led back to the car. It was almost as if I was in a trance.

Deep down I knew it was not over, although for now the aggression had left him. But I knew he had not finished with me yet.

I sat still, my head hung low as he started to drive again. In a soft voice, the kind of voice someone would use if they were having a chilled out chat over a cup of coffee, the questions came.

'How long has this been going on? How long have you been seeing him? Was he a good fuck? Did you enjoy it?'

I knew once again that it would not matter what I said. The same questions were asked over and over again. He was getting more and more aggressive as he asked them. He was screaming now, 'ANSWER ME YOU SLAG.'

He suddenly stopped the car and was on top of me, beating me again, my head pressed against the window as he repeatedly punched me, every punch matching the syllable of each word. I felt every hit but I also felt numb. I sat there and took it, for I had learned years ago that fighting against him would only make it worse, make him more angry. It wasn't long before he tired of this and kicked me out of the car. He drove off again.

Now, my only thought was that if he had come back once, he would come back again. I had to get up. I had to get off the road. My body hurt and physically all I wanted to do was lie there. I was breathing heavily and my ribs hurt with every breath. I began to talk to myself, 'Get up. Get up. Get out of here now.' I felt hate and anger for him and fear that if I didn't get out now he would be back. So I got up and I got off the road and went into a field, wanting to be as far away from him as possible and out of his sight. I knew that if I didn't get out of this now I would never get out of it. He would kill me, and if I'm honest with myself, if I went back, I would probably have let him kill me.

That night I managed through sheer determination to get away. Somehow I got to my friend David's and after a few phone calls and a little bit of organising I was on a coach. It was not the worst beating he had given me, but it was the last.

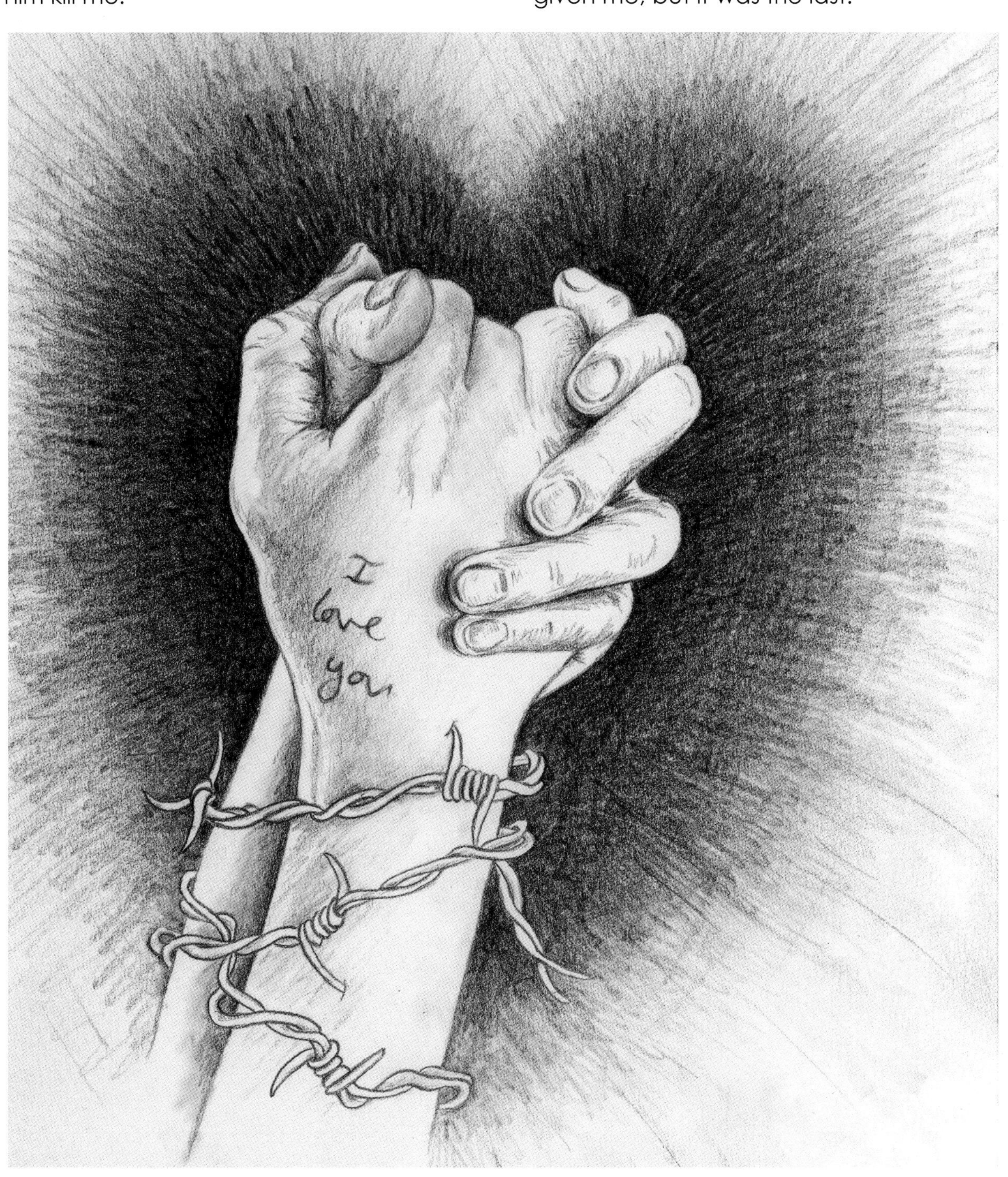

The phone call

December 2012

'Hello.'

And there it was. That voice that had a way of making me feel instant fear. Saying one simple word that almost made my heart stop, my body stiffen. It was him after all this time. What could he want? Why was he ringing? All these thoughts went through my mind in that split second from hearing his voice. Trying to hide the panic in my voice, I hesitantly answered.

'Hi.'

'How are you?'

'Err. I'm OK thanks. How are you?'

'Long time no hear!' he said casually as if he was talking to an old friend and not the woman he had beaten on so many occasions. The woman who he had nearly succeeded in destroying. The woman who gave up everything and moved over 250 miles away – just to get away from him.

'Yes. I hope you don't mind me ringing. I just thought I would say "Hello".'

'Oh OK.'

'Can you talk? Have I rung at a bad time?'

'No, it's fine. So how's life?'

'I had a fight the other day. Some prick started on me. But you know how it is. I showed them. Oh and me and Gemma have split up.'

And there it was. Right there. The whole reason he was ringing me. Gemma was the other woman who he had been seeing behind my back for nearly a year. Just one of many. So he had finished with her, had he? But was he really that dense? Did he really expect me to go running back to him, now?

Well where do I start? It's been non-stop for me. I've passed my English. Oh, and I've sold a couple of drawings.

'Oh dear. What happened?' I faked interest.

'She's twisted. She's accused me of rape. I'm a lot of things but I'm no rapist!'

'Oh no. That's awful Rob.' I said, feigning sympathy.

'Yeah. The police know it's all bullshit. She's dirty scum. Anyway, how's things with you? What have you been up to?'

'Well where do I start?' I began. 'It's been non-stop for me. I've been studying. I've passed my English. Oh, and I've sold a couple of my drawings. I've made some lovely friends. Oh yeah, and I'm having some of my writing published...'

Oh wow. How good this was feeling. His voice changed instantly, not to anger, but I could hear in the tone, he was gutted, totally gutted that I was doing so well.

'Oh great,' he said, but I could hear the jealousy in his voice, and before he had the chance to say anything I carried on.

'Oh Rob, my life is great. I'm doing really well. Moving away was the best thing I've ever done. Anyway I've got to go. Take care. Bye.'

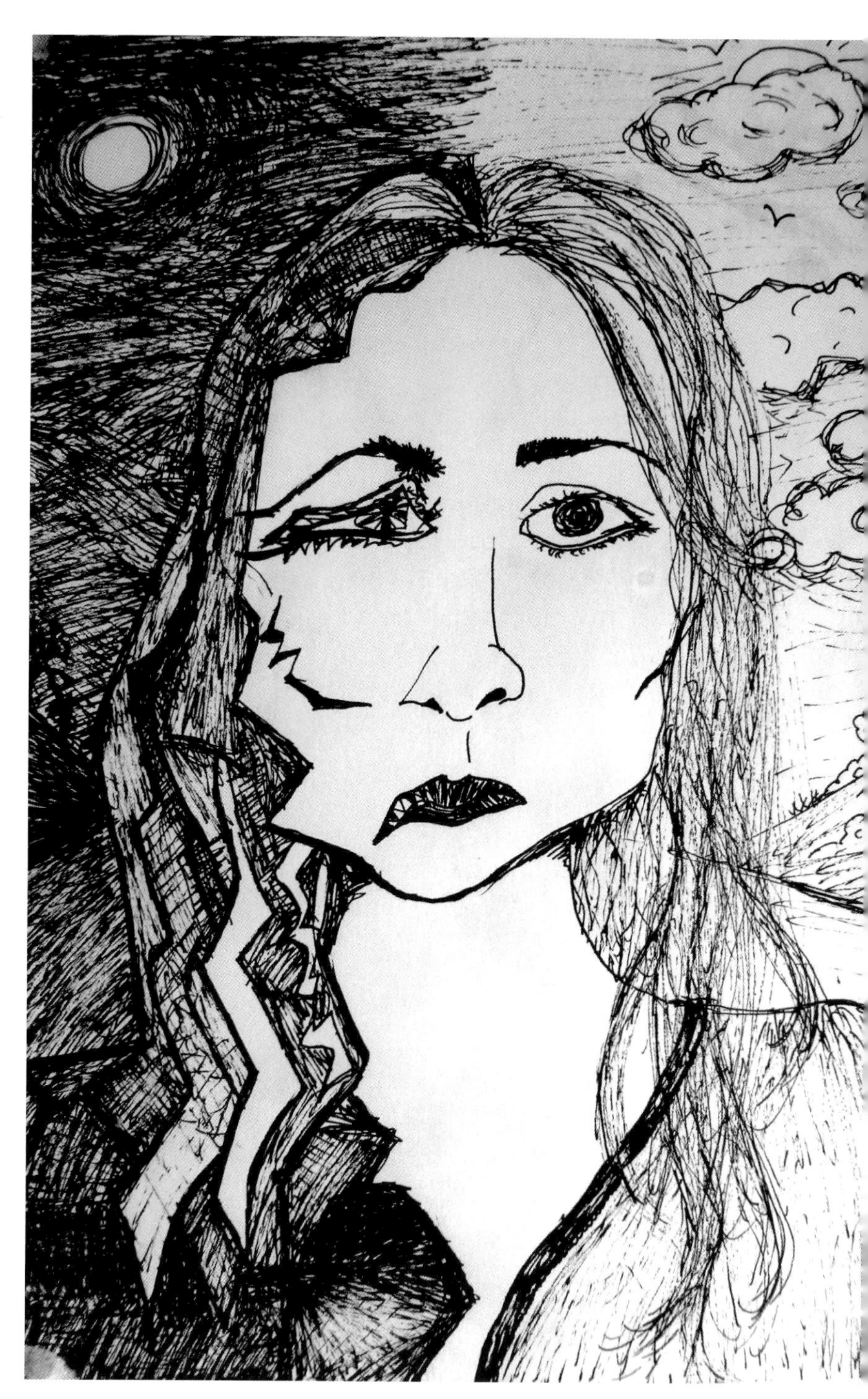

And there it was. Our conversation was over. I had the biggest smile of satisfaction on my face. Just being able to say how good my life was. It was empowering. For the first time since I had known him, I wasn't that weak person under his control. I finally had the upper hand and it was better than any argument or slanging match that we could have got into. Just the fact that I was doing well and my life hadn't crumbled hurt him more than any harsh words could ever have done.

He's tried calling a few times since then, but I've ignored him.

My life has changed.

I'm free.

I'm free from his control, free to speak to who I want to without the fear of being beaten, free to wear what I want to wear, go where I want to go.

Free to be me.

You are not alone

May 2013

If you are in a similar situation and can relate to these stories, I hope that they have shown you that you are not alone. You don't know how strong you are until being strong is your only choice. Finding the strength to leave when I did saved my life.

During the two years leading up to finally leaving him I started getting myself strong. I attended groups for women in domestic abusive relationships. At the time, I didn't feel they helped me as I was made to attend them by the local authorities and I didn't have a good attitude towards them. But they started to make me see Rob in a different light. I began to disassociate myself from him and gradually realised he was an abuser and a control freak on many levels. Even though it still took me a long time to finally leave him, I came away from those groups with a lot of knowledge and tips about how to live safely with an abuser. They also made me realise that I wasn't alone and that there were many women out there living in the same sort of circumstances as me. So, although they felt useless at the time, they really did help me.

I began to disassociate myself from him and gradually realised he was an abuser...

When I first came to Exeter I would probably have gone back to him after a couple of days if it wasn't for my friend David. He got me to contact an old friend, Sandra, who I hadn't seen for years. We stayed with her and I realised just how much they were prepared to help. I would never have thought of bothering them or asking for help but between them they convinced me to stay for a bit longer. No, not convinced, they confirmed what I had known for a long time, that Rob was dangerous and that he would never change. I thought my stay should only be for a couple of weeks. I had a flat and animals to get back to. It was only ever going to be a break, just a bit of time to get my head straight, to have a think. I never imagined that I would never go back. But the fact that I was now over 250 miles away and had put that distance between us, really helped me to find the time to grow strong enough to end the relationship for good. That, and the fact that he kept ringing me, one minute begging me to come back and the next threatening me. Being so far away and knowing he wasn't around the corner, even though I did miss him a lot in the beginning, made it so much easier for me to end it.

My first six months were hard and quite scary. I was drinking really heavily, up to nine litres of strong cider a day. I think it was a coping mechanism.

Christmas time was the hardest. I was away from my family and friends and everything I had ever known. I missed my children terribly. On the outside looking in, everything was fine, but I had got so good at living a lie. I was a master of disguise.

I was living in a bedsit while the council decided if they were going to help me or not. They decided they wouldn't and this was the last straw. I was scared of the prospect of having to return. Rob was still threatening me and if I returned I knew I would have ended up back in his clutches. And I knew the beatings would be worse than ever.

I lost all hope and I attempted suicide. I took an overdose. I don't remember much about it and I moved into The Esther Community straight from the hospital. This was also scary at first. I had never lived with so many women. But it wasn't as scary as I thought. Suddenly, I wasn't alone. I got stronger over the months, I made some wonderful friends and I even started getting an education. I started to feel like a part of society and I began to discover who I was after all those years. I joined a creative writing class and met a wonderful and amazing teacher and became part of a close-knit group. I began to write about my experiences. This has helped me unbelievably towards recovery. Writing about the beatings he gave me and reading it in black and white made me really realise just how bad it actually was. This cemented in my head why I could never go back.

On the outside looking in, everything was fine, but I had got so good at living a lie. I was a master of disguise.

I don't drink every day any more. I'm not one hundred percent better but I'm getting there. What I have been through isn't an easy fix, but The Esther Community has helped me so much and my wonderful writing group has given me something positive to focus on.

I've made a lot of mistakes. I have upset my family and failed my children. Sometimes the guilt is almost crippling. But I won't give up and I want to prove to the people I love that I have changed. I have achieved more in this past year than I did in all my years at school. I'm finally learning to be me again and to stop punishing myself for my past mistakes. I am learning to accept the choices I have made and to concentrate on my future.

Writing about the beatings... made me really realise just how bad it actually was.

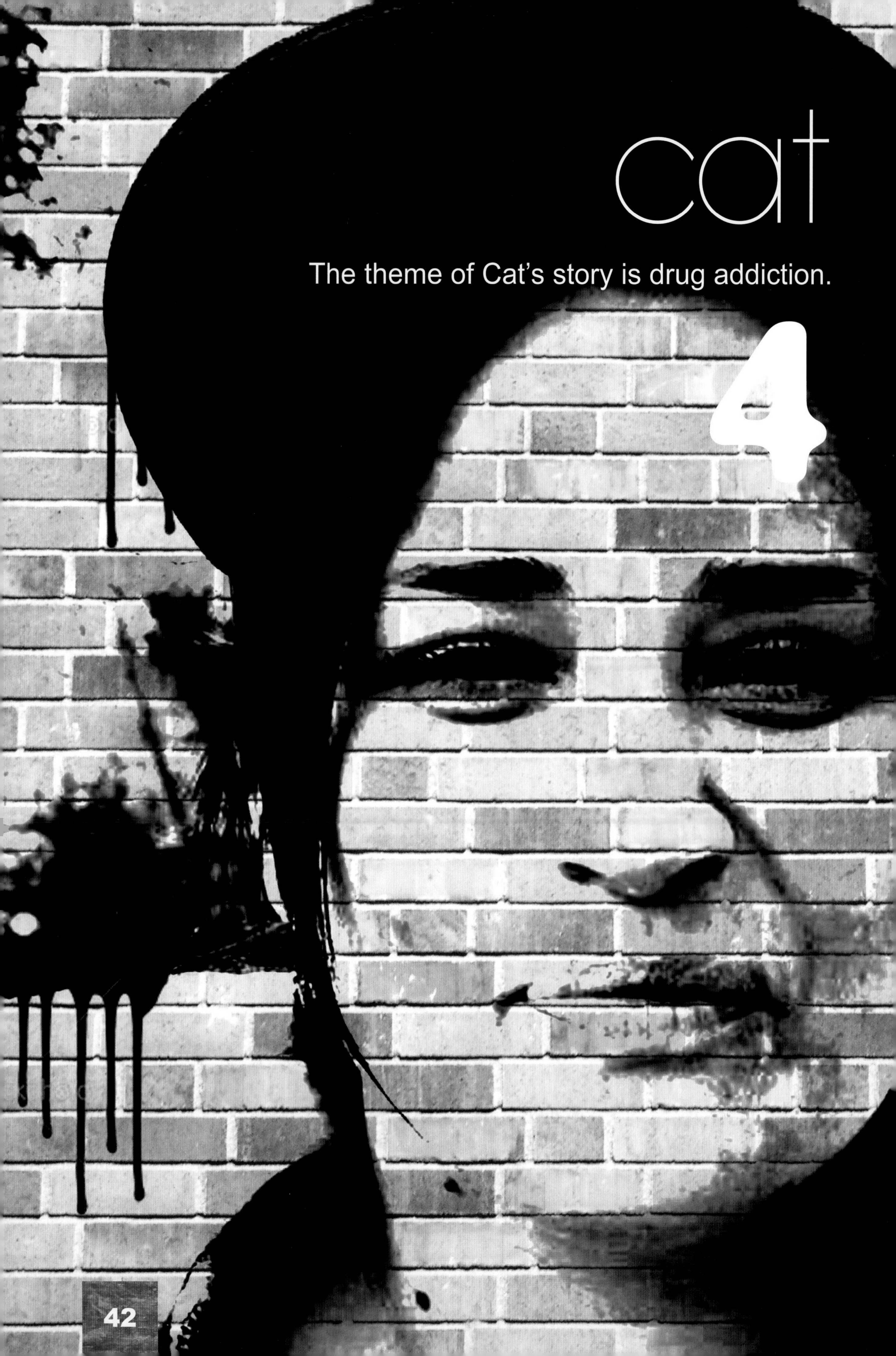

cat

The theme of Cat's story is drug addiction.

4

my story

I grew up in a small village in North Wales surrounded by a big extended family. When I was ten my father got a job in Exeter and we moved into a new home in what seemed to be a massive city.

I did really well at school and was academically two years above my age. But I became very bored, and when I was eleven, I started experimenting with different drugs. I was quite shy at that time but I soon discovered that drugs gave me power and confidence. By the time I was sixteen I was addicted to heroin and crack cocaine. This was followed by a succession of drug-related prison sentences. For ten years I detached myself from my family and moved to Bristol. It was there that I started prostitution in order to fund my habit.

During that time I injected into a vein in my shin which became a venous ulcer. This has got progressively worse and I have been admitted into hospital for treatment at least fifteen times in the last ten years. I am still battling with it today.

I returned to Exeter at the age of thirty to try and get clean and stay off drugs. I'm still on that journey now and hope to go to a residential rehab.

I enjoy the use of English and words and I aspire to be a lyricist.

A lot to lose

September 2001

The sound of police sirens. This was not unusual in my area but there were a lot of them so I put down my crack pipe and snuck over to the window to check out what was happening. As I looked out I noticed Yankee, a dealer who lived in the same block as me, trying to bury a plastic bag in the garden. Immediately I knew that it was his stash and he was putting it away for the night. I didn't really think much of it as I already had drugs of my own, but as usual they didn't last very long.

I was twenty years old and I lived and breathed for drugs. Drugs made me feel invincible and I would take as much of anything and everything as I could. I had lost my family because of drugs and so drugs and all they stood for became my family. They were always there for me as long as I could earn enough money to pay for them, which I always could. I worked a street in a well-known red light district in Bristol and I could earn as much money as I needed. I was a bad girl and I loved being known and respected for it. I took ridiculous risks. I would get into complete strangers' cars and let them take me to the middle of nowhere, not even knowing where I was going, and then let them do whatever they wanted to me. I would be out on the street 24/7, until I couldn't stay awake anymore. And all for drugs. I didn't care about anything apart from drugs. Live or die as long as I was high.

I was twenty years old and I lived and breathed for drugs

So, after smoking my last piece of crack I had a thought. I would just go down to the garden and dig up Yankee's stash so I could get high again. I sat and deliberated for all of sixty seconds and then proceeded to search for tools. All I could find after my search of the flat was a kitchen fork, so I put my cap on, pulled my hoody on tight and did a James Bond to the garden. I didn't feel at all guilty about this as I had spent over £2,000 with this dealer. But my heart was in my mouth in case he caught me in the act. I knew I was being really reckless this time and I knew if he caught me I would be beaten up, stabbed or raped. This was complete madness, but I was so used to taking risks, and I wanted those drugs.

When I got there, I began frantically stabbing the ground with the fork in the spot where I was pretty sure it was. With each stab of the ground, unbeknown to me, I was piercing holes into the bag. After ten minutes of searching I eventually found my prize. It was a good find, almost half of heroin and half of crack, worth £1,500. I was literally the cat who got the cream! I actually felt like I'd won the lottery on a rollover week. I quickly hid the bag in my jacket but was too paranoid to go back to my flat in case he had an idea it was me. So I decided to go to the nearest multi-storey car park to prepare the biggest hit of heroin and crack I could fit into a needle. The car park was about five storeys high and I went right up to the top level. There were little lights at the top of each stairway and I sat down directly underneath the last one to cook up my hit. This car park was used a lot by addicts and I was panicking at the thought of someone seeing me. All addicts tend to know each other or know someone who you score off and I was really worried that someone would come up the stairway and see me with all these drugs and start asking questions. I knew I could easily blag it and say I had robbed a punter but I still didn't want Yankee getting even the slightest hint that I had been near a lot of drugs. Addicts are the worst grasses I have ever met. Offer them a hit and they will tell you anything! I was so paranoid but I still carried on. It was dark in the car park and even though I was sitting underneath a light, I couldn't see the particles of soil that had mixed in with the powder. But, even if I had, I wouldn't have cared because all I wanted to do was to get off my head.

I didn't have an inkling how much damage this one hit would do to my life.

But to my shock and horror, each week the wound got larger and larger. The doctor blamed it on my continuous use of drugs...

Three months down the line I developed a small raw patch over the injection site. I just assumed it would get better, but I was kidding myself. I started to go the doctor's every week to have my leg checked and the wound cleaned. But to my shock and horror, each week the wound got larger and larger. The doctor blamed it on my continuous use of drugs and also explained that the drugs I had stolen that night had been contaminated by the soil. I had a venous ulcer.

Over the next eleven years I have continued to use drugs and the ulcer now covers the whole of the bottom of my leg, back and front. Daily I go through the horror of having the wounds cleaned and dressed. The doctors are still saying it will eventually improve but may take up to twenty years. I feel I am in an impossible situation as although I now desperately want to stay off drugs, I am in so much pain from my ulcer; I keep going back to them to take the pain away. I know that by continuing to use drugs I am preventing the healing process and I don't know how long I can continue like this.

I am now using every agency available to me to try and deal with the consequences of my actions on that day in September 2001. I am not giving up.

Paradise manifest

You see I loved hard drugs,
But the love was unreturned.
I found out without no doubt
Ain't nobody was concerned.
In time it turned.

Drugs tried to burn me.
And though my eyes saw the deception
My heart wouldn't let me learn.
Some dumb woman was I
'Cos every time I'd lie
Inside I'd die.

My heart must've died a thousand deaths.
Compared myself to Toni Braxton.
Thought I'd never catch my breath.
NOTHING LEFT.

Drugs stole the heart beating in my chest.
I tried to call the cops.
But that type of thief they can't arrest.
Pain suppressed will lead to cardiac arrest.

I was God's blessed.
Spent nights with my arms across
my chest,
Contemplating death with a Gillette.
But NO DRUG is ever worth
A PARADISE MANIFEST.

I used to love her

As I look at what I've done
This hyper life that I have lived.
How many things I've prayed
Father would forgive.

There was a young woman.
She was the ocean
And I was the sand.
She stole my heart
Like a thief in the night,
Troubled my senses
And worried my mind.
But I used to love her.

Torn and confused
Wasted and used
Reached a crossroads.
Which path would I choose?
Stuck and frustrated
I waited, debated
For something to change.

My heart was deflated
Thought what I wanted
Was something I needed
When Mamma said, 'No!'
Then I just should've heeded
That night I bled
'Til the poison was gone
And now I've spat that
I must be done!

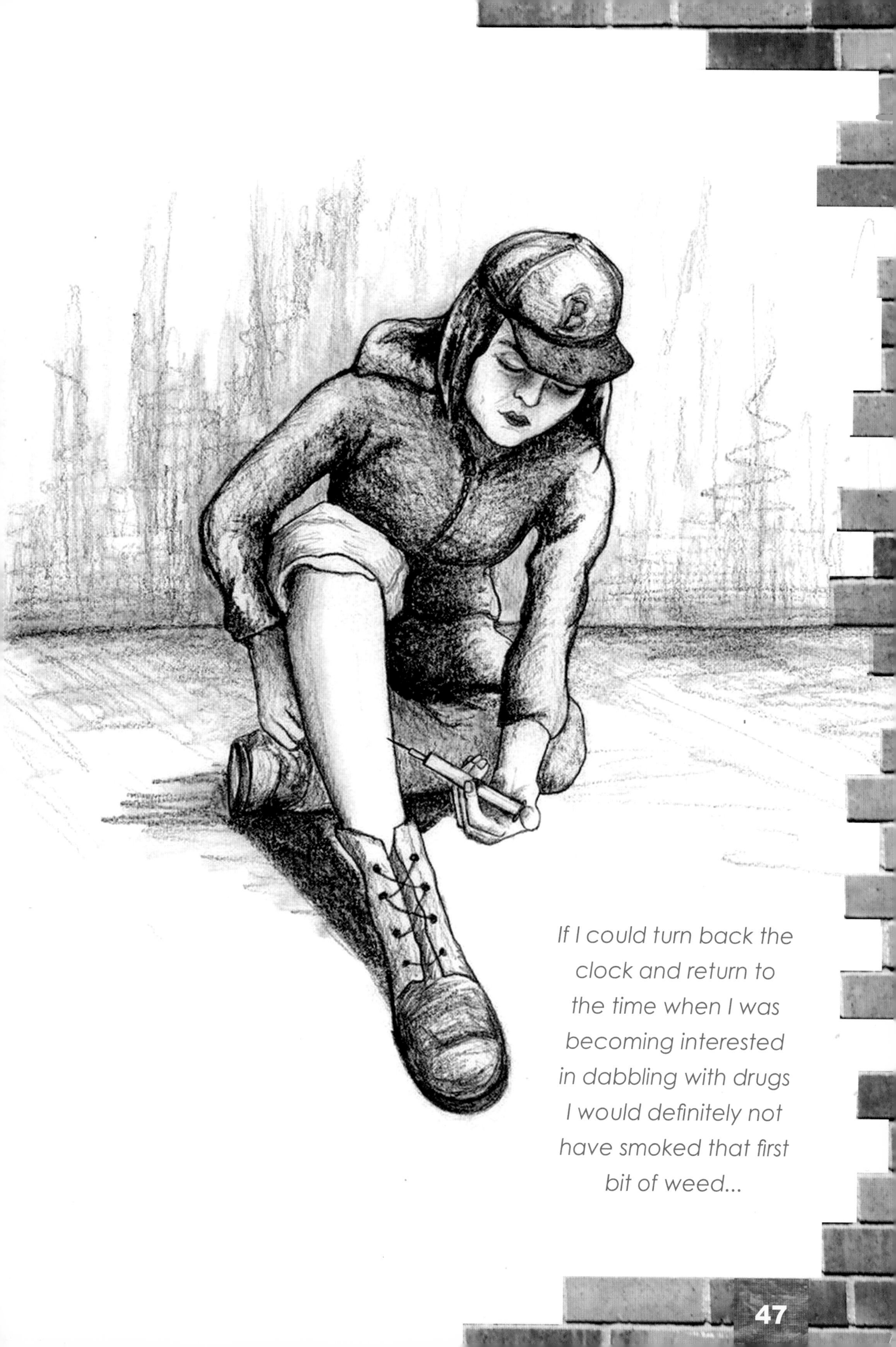
If I could turn back the
clock and return to
the time when I was
becoming interested
in dabbling with drugs
I would definitely not
have smoked that first
bit of weed...

A slap in the face

January 2013

The last three weeks had been hell on earth. But I had managed to get through them and was now free from the shackles of daily heroin use. I'd achieved this almost impossible feat by hibernating and isolating myself from all other addicts. I was so jealous of them being off their heads, I just couldn't face them. But it was also physically, emotionally and psychologically very, very hard. I found just having to deal with anything, without being totally wrecked, was hard. Even simple things like walking into the smoking room and talking to my friends was hard. All my confidence had suddenly gone. Drugs gave me the confidence to be who I was, to be Cat, but now I couldn't even look friends in the eye, let alone have a proper conversation with them. I was turning back into that shy thirteen-year-old girl without any drugs in her, and I didn't know how to cope. But nevertheless, I was at least drug free.

I had worked so hard to stay clean and to be given this chance to change my life forever.

Thursday morning arrived and I was in the grip of terror and excitement, for today I was going to visit a residential rehab. I had worked so hard to stay clean and to be given this chance to change my life forever. I awoke on auto-pilot and got dressed in my best clothes, applied make-up and perfume and even got my hair straightened. I wanted to make a good impression. At 9.30 am my drug worker picked me up and I got into his car together with my support worker from the hostel.

'You sure want to make a good impression, don't you?' he remarked as we started our journey.

'What, because you've never seen me look so together?' I replied, feeling slightly hurt, but I really did want him to see how much I could pull myself together, if I needed to. I was in jokey mode and as usual, I acted the clown, but inside I was full of fear and trepidation.

When we arrived the manager greeted us with a cheery smile. She was not what I was expecting. She was of the hippy generation, dressed in hippy gear with long red hair and loads of beads. She grabbed my hand and shook it wholeheartedly.

'You must be Kate,' she stated. This already felt weird as I hated being called Kate and I realised that if I entered into this programme for real that was who I would have to be! Lots of people in authority wanted me to lose the nickname Cat. They thought that Cat was my alter ego (the addict) so they were all determined to call me Kate.

She then gave us a tour of the whole building and she was positive and upbeat about the whole programme. The building was gorgeous but I felt quite out of my depth. She explained that because of my leg I would have to have a longer detox and a different regime than the other addicts. I felt very worried and unsure about this, particularly as I knew the pain in my leg would increase if I didn't have the methadone to numb it. How would I manage? As I was thinking about this a patient came out of her room. She was the only patient I met that day and she looked absolutely terrible. She was half-way through her methadone detox and she was crying and apologising profusely to the manager about being late for a group therapy session. She said she hadn't slept for weeks and as she talked she retched into a sick bowl that she was carrying. I realised suddenly that she was the embodiment of my worst fears of a methadone detox. Now, I was having very mixed feelings. I could almost see me coming out of that room saying the same things, except I would be in agony with my leg too. It was horrible. On the one hand, I wanted to be clean and have a 'normal' life but I didn't want to go through what that girl was going through. We walked on and the manager went on to talk about how great the bedrooms were, but would I really care about that if I was climbing the walls? I realised then that this place was in fact a beautiful nightmare.

During the journey back I was silent and shell-shocked. I didn't talk about how I felt as I didn't want my drug worker to know just how terrified I was.

On arrival back at the hostel I was greeted with a barrage of questions and accusations. But not about my visit. One of the residents had removed the washing that I had put on for me and my friend early that morning before I left for Plymouth. On emptying the machine she had discovered a needle... and told the staff. I couldn't believe it. It had nothing to do with me. But I knew my friend could be in very serious trouble. She had already had a number of warnings. So I just decided there and then to be loyal to her and tell them that it was my needle. But I also knew that this was a perfect way out of having to go to rehab. The staff would have to tell my drug worker, and I would be off the hook.

I realised suddenly that she was the embodiment of my worst fears of a methadone detox.

I walked into town, feeling happy with my decision, and found my friend. After all my efforts to become, and remain, clean, I gave into the reality that I didn't have the strength for everything that normality entailed.

'Hey babe, look, don't freak out on me but someone found the pin in your washing and told the staff,' I said, feeling anxious and not wanting to cause an argument.

'You said you would get it out,' she barked back.

'Yeah I know but while I was out someone else found it. I'm sorry.'

'So that's me out then, init?'

'No, coz I told the staff it was my washing too, so they'll think it's mine,' I said.

'Seriously Cat, did you? Coz you know I'm on my last warning, don't you?'

'Yes, I promise. Come on. You know I'm

always there for you. I would never let you down.'

I was trying desperately to reassure her as I could see that she was really panicking but at the same time she seemed so ungrateful for what I had done and then all she wanted to know was did I have any money for drugs. She didn't even ask me how my day had gone. MY BIG DAY. I felt so hurt, but even so, I went to the cash point and took some money out and gave it to her. She said she would get drugs for both of us.

I went home and waited for her to come back but she didn't. She finally returned two nights later, having spent all my money on drugs for herself. I was devastated. She didn't even apologise. This was a major slap in the face for me. I thought we were really good friends, really close, but I was forced to accept that no matter how close a friendship you think you have, drugs will come before anything and everything.

The next day I went back to my emotional crutch and physical saviour – drugs. What a mistake that was. When will I learn my lesson?

Not giving up

June 2013

Although I'm still on my journey to complete recovery and abstinence from drugs I feel that I have come a long way since the time I spent in Bristol. My last prison sentence was for two street robberies, and for those crimes I received four and a half years. In that time I grew up a lot and had plenty of time to reflect on how much of a mess my life was in. It also quickly became clear who my friends were. I can honestly say that there were only two people that stood by me during that sentence. Those two people are still in my life now and are constantly encouraging me to improve myself. It's often said by addicts that no one is your friend, you only have acquaintances. This has certainly been the reality for me.

It's often said by addicts that no one is your friend, you only have acquaintances.

I returned to Exeter to my family and tried repeatedly to stay off drugs. Even though I ended up running back to them when I was hurt, scared, worried or upset, there were still periods in my life when I used just the medication I was prescribed. That in itself was one of the biggest battles I faced. I had been on methadone and diazepam since I was fourteen years old.

While I was living in The Esther Community I was really helped by the support of family and friends. I loved having a laugh with my friends and I think the giggles we used to have helped me take my mind off the pain in my leg. There is a lot to be said for the power of laughter. I also gained a lot by joining the creative writing class. I was able to be myself in those classes and I loved being able to sit down and achieve something, as apart from getting high, I hadn't achieved anything in the whole of my life. I tried some sessions at N.A. (Narcotics Anonymous) and while it was great knowing that I wasn't alone, I didn't feel they worked for me, as all we did was talk about how bad drugs were, and I didn't really see the point in that as I already knew, all too well, just how bad they were.

If I could turn back the clock and return to the time when I was becoming interested in dabbling with drugs I would definitely not have smoked that first bit of weed – let alone picked up that needle full of heroin and crack and injected it into my system. I have lost everything through using drugs. It stole my family from me, robbed me of an education and, worst of all, my health has deteriorated badly. I wish that children in schools were taught the realities of drug use and introduced to someone like me.

I have now left The Esther Community and Exeter and moved away from the area in order to distance myself from other addicts and try again to sort my life out. I miss my family. They have always been supportive of me but it was only when I grew up that I realised that they were using tough love as a way of protecting themselves and to help me realise that it's only me who can get clean for me. I have to do it for myself, not for them.

Now I need to really persevere to stay off drugs and get my leg healed. Then I would love to go to a residential rehab. I need to learn the life skills that I didn't learn when I was younger but I also know that I will need an immense amount of will power.

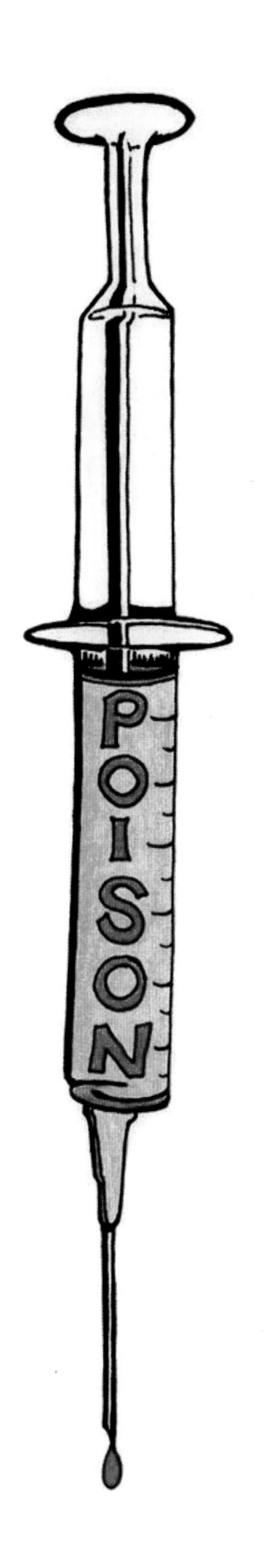

emma m.

The theme of Emma M's story is homelessness.

5

my story

I grew up in a small town called Nairn in the Highlands of Scotland. My family moved there when I was five years old but I never felt that I fitted in very well. I was always a loner and, as soon as I turned fifteen, I left for London, where I became involved in drink and drugs and eventually became homeless.

I left London when I was twenty and moved to the Isle of Skye where I got married and had a son. The marriage broke down after a few years and I moved to Exeter to live with my sister. I had another unsuccessful relationship and had a daughter. I lived on the straight and narrow for a while, but eventually drink and drugs crept back into my life and I became homeless again. My daughter went to live with other family members. I was homeless on and off for four years. I have lived in tents, car-park stairwells and hostels. I am now living in a B&B.

I don't have any high aspirations. I would like to live a normal life, working in a paid job and be able to see my children and be a mother again.

Trapped

April 2010

Rudely awoken by a nudge in my side, I opened my eyes and had to blink away the bright sunlight that was filtering into our cream-coloured tent. I could tell he was in a bad mood. He always was in the morning. I heard him getting dressed and unzipping the tent so he could spit out of the gap, something that always annoyed me. Then came the smoker's cough and the hacking, phlegmy noises. 'Charming,' I thought.

'Come on! Get up. We need to get some money together to score,' he barked.

'Yeah, okay, in a minute,' I said sleepily.

'No. Now! Sooner we go on the rob, the sooner we get better.' He pulled the covers off me which he knew I hated.

'I don't want to get up. I can't do this anymore. I would rather go without gear than go through another day of stealing. I can't do it anymore. I am tired and stressed out from all the traipsing around that we have to do every day.'

I felt so isolated now that I was homeless and living in a tent. It was like the world was carrying on without me and didn't care about me.

I really was an emotional wreck. I felt so isolated now that I was homeless and living in a tent. It was like the world was carrying on without me and didn't care about me. Then again, I didn't care about myself anymore either. I was just a useless junkie who deserved this sorry excuse of a life. All I wanted to do was lie in the tent and not see anybody. My confidence was at an all time low, especially as my kids were now in the care of my family because of my chronic alcoholism and bad choice in men. I just wanted to curl up and forget the world. I yanked the covers back up over my head and lay really still, hoping that he would forget I was there and go without me. I heard him rummaging around, looking for his tobacco and matches.

'You'd better be up and dressed before I've smoked my rollie – or I'll drag you out instead,' he said moodily. As I knew he was capable of doing just that, I slowly got up and started pulling on my damp clothes. I noticed that they were starting to smell and had ingrained dirt on the knees. I had never felt so unclean and unkempt. I had always taken pride in my appearance, but now I just felt like a tramp. I crawled out of the tent and stepped into my trainers, which were still wet from the rain the night before.

'Yuk! They are soaking,' I mumbled.

'Oh stop moaning for God's sake,' he snapped. 'You're never happy. Why are you so negative all the time?' I didn't bother to answer as he never understood what I had lost. He never would.

'Well I'm ready now, so let's go. But can't we just try and get clean from now on?' I asked. 'I can't go on like this babe. We could be doing a lot more with our lives. Get jobs again. I really am going to have a nervous breakdown soon. I can feel my head about to explode. Please don't make me keep stealing.' I looked at him imploringly, hoping he would see how near to breaking point I was.

All I got was a scowl and told to, 'Move your ass now.' We got our bags together, zipped up the tent and started our twenty-five minute walk through mud-soaked paths into town. There was a silence that you could cut through with a knife. I was deep in thought and he was just plain moody.

As we neared the town he said, 'We'll get some wine from the Co-op first, then go sell it for some gear.'

'Can we not have some breakfast first? I'm really hungry,' I asked.

'No. I will nick you a sandwich or something. I need a hit first. Now stop being so selfish.'

Maybe I was selfish for wanting to eat instead of helping graft for money, for drugs.

I really had to fight back the tears that were welling up. My eyes stung and my face felt hot and flushed. My head started hurting with the pure frustration of it all. Was I over-reacting? Maybe I was selfish for wanting to eat instead of helping graft for money, for drugs. For the millionth time, I bit my tongue and nodded in agreement. There was never any point in arguing anyway.

As we approached the shop, I felt the usual knot in my stomach as my nerves addled away. What if we got caught this time? I couldn't handle being locked up in a cell for most of the day. Then again, at least I would get fed. We walked in and towards the alcohol section. We never spoke and I opened my bag and he handed me four bottles of wine, one by one in quick succession. I put them in my bag. I kept a look out and as I couldn't fit any more in, he put two bottles into his coat. Then he pretended his phone was ringing and that was our cue to walk out of the shop. I must admit there was a certain rush once we had got out of the shop and up the end of the road. A kind of exhilaration knowing we were half-way to scoring. All we had to do now was sell the wine, then score some gear.

Once we got the money, we walked through town to see what dealer we could find. Along the way we met a few people who were also looking to buy some heroin but told us that everyone they had phoned had run out. There was a dry spell. It was horrible when there was none around. After more and more dead ends, we decided to just rob some more alcohol so we could have a drink instead.

So, back to the shop we trudged and repeated the routine of robbery. This time, he picked up some sherry, which was always a bad combination with him, especially as he was in a really bad mood by now. As I watched him glug it down, I had the sense of on-coming trouble. He had that look in his eyes that appeared when he was out of his head, which always ended up in tears. Mine first, then his the next day, when he was begging for forgiveness for stuff he couldn't remember saying or doing the night or day before.

I decided that I would go back to the tent as I was still tired and in desperate need of sleep. I did not for one minute think that this would be a problem as he seemed quite happy swigging away at the sherry.

'Hey babe. I'm gonna go back to the tent as there is not much point in wandering about town with no money,' I said.

'No, you can't. We may as well rob some perfume while we're in town so we can sell it when someone turns up with some gear. Come on. We'll go to Boots and try.'

I shook my head and started to walk the other way back towards the tent.

'No. I am going for a sleep but I am not stopping you from staying in town. See you when you get back. Just be careful. OK.' I went to kiss him goodbye but he jerked his head away and glared at me.

'You stay with ME. We have got to stick together.'

I tried to remind him that we were not joined at the hip and we were allowed some time apart. I started to walk away from him. I got as far as a couple of metres when all of a sudden I felt his hand grab my arm roughly, pulling me back towards him. When I turned my head round, his eyes were full of hatred and he was bright red from the effects of the sherry. I tried to pull my arm away but he was too strong and was now pushing me against the hard brick wall of the supermarket, pinning me up by my neck. As I struggled, he held me tighter and thrust his knee up against me so hard I could not move at all. It was all happening in what seemed like slow motion, yet people that were passing by seemed to speed up and I could not, and would not, look into their eyes in fear that they might try and help, which would only end up with more of a scene and violence.

I was aware of children walking closer to their parents, and I was thinking how lucky it was that they were kept safe and hopefully never had to witness violence like this in their family. I thought how I should have done more to try and prevent my own kids from seeing their mother being strangled and pulled about by her hair, kicked when she was down. All of these thoughts went through my head. The hurt, the guilt, the tears and the pain after all those months of abuse, welled up in me like a volcano about to erupt. I could feel the fury inside of me firing up, ready to explode out of my soul, wanting to destroy this demonic monster that had such a bitter, twisted hold on me. I hated him so much at that moment.

He was now shouting in my face but all I could do was stand there, numb with fury, watching his mouth wording horrible, nasty comments and names. Then I just felt myself snap. I started to push him away with all the strength I could muster.

I shouted, 'Get the hell away from me. I hate you so much and don't love you anymore. You are a twat and I wish I had never met you. Leave me the fuck alone.'

His eyes glazed over but instead of letting me go, he tightened his stranglehold and with a sneer, spat straight on my face. I couldn't believe it: the ultimate insult. I could not hear what he was saying anymore as I was in shock from how quickly he had turned on me. My knees buckled and I slid down the wall as he finally let go of my neck. There was a man shouting from across the road, telling him to leave me alone. All the poor

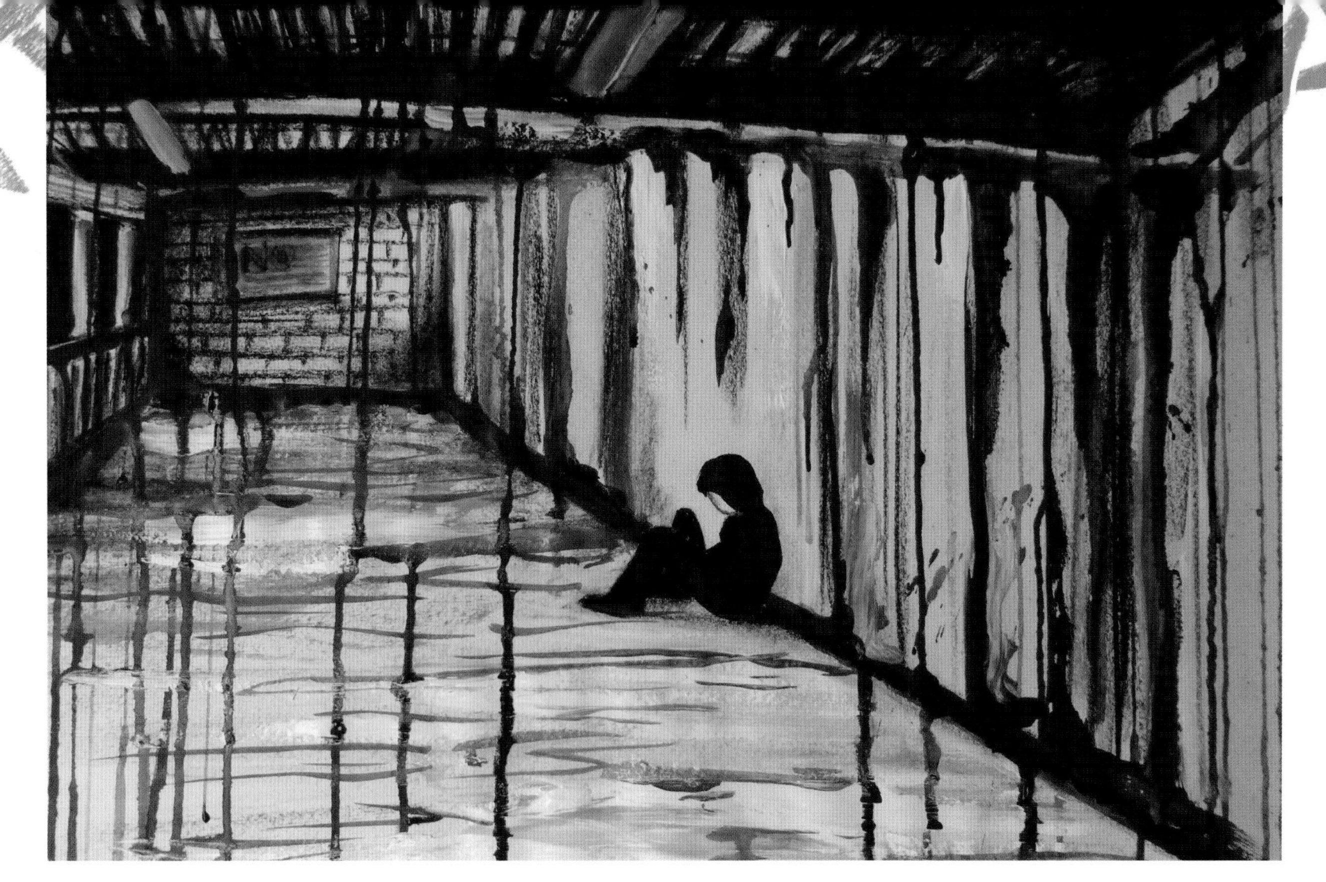

man got in return for his concern for me, was a rude, 'Do one Twat.'

As he turned round towards the road, I ripped myself from the wall and ran as fast as I could up the road and towards the nearest pub. I was aware of the spit dripping off my clothes. I rubbed it away furiously with the sleeve of my coat. He was starting to run behind me but I got to the pub entrance first and ran into the bar, full of old men nursing their half-pints. They looked up at me as I walked gingerly up to the bar to ask where the toilets were. As the landlady pointed over to the ladies' toilets, I spotted him hovering outside. He was too much of a coward to come into a pub full of people, which was a huge relief. I could relax for a moment and go and clean my face and coat. I went into the toilet cubicle and sat down, my head in my hands. I was breathing heavily and my heart was still pounding. I realised I was shaking like a leaf. I thought I was going to pass out.

I sat for a bit and thought about what to do next. Now was my chance to get rid of him for good. I didn't need him and I sure hated him right now. I was fed up with the drunken rants and the violent episodes. I wanted to get my life back in order and get my kids back. If only I could get him to stop drinking then our lives would be perfect. I loved his sober side. In truth, I loved him more than any other man I had been with. He did take care of me after all.

I suddenly realised I was back-pedalling and making excuses for his behaviour. Who was I kidding? I was always going to go back to him. There was a spark in the beginning and there would be till the end.

So I left the toilet cubicle and stood looking at myself in the mirror. I looked like a different woman entirely. I had bags under my eyes and my hair was greasy from not being washed in so long. I splashed some water onto my tear-streaked face and then left the sanctuary of that dingy toilet and smoke-stained pub.

He was waiting a few metres down the road and as I approached him he held out his hand and as I took it he pulled me to him and hugged me hard.

'Come on, babe, let's go,' he murmured.

Rock bottom

October 2011

Can you remember your first childhood dreams and aspirations? Did they involve a life married to the perfect person and living in your very own dream home? Or were you going to travel the globe and help save this beautiful planet?

At the age of ten, my vision of the future all seemed so simple. All I had to do was get a job after attending university with my best friend, who I would share an apartment with whilst studying nursing, as I had always wanted to help people in need. After we graduated from university we would then meet our respective boyfriends and get married – a double wedding of course, because we were best friends and we would always be together.

I can remember waiting excitedly for my mother's shopping catalogue to arrive so that my sister and I could look through it together and choose new clothes. We would sit side by side on the living room floor and thumb through it, choosing items of furniture that we would buy for our new homes once we had married and had children. We had a game that we would play where we were not allowed to choose the same items as each other and we had to pick at least one thing from each page. My favourite section was the mother and baby clothing and accessories. I enjoyed choosing cute little romper suits and cot bedding which would suit the decor of our nursery bedroom. I always vowed that if I had a little girl I would not paint her room pink but different tones of purple and turquoise. Oh, the excitement of it all!

How impatient I was to 'grow up' and be able to buy whatever I wanted. Life seemed so black and white. I would be able to do anything and everything because I would be an adult and have a job that paid for my glorious, happy and carefree lifestyle.

So why had I ended up sat in a dirty shop doorway, homeless, and drinking a tin of super-strength lager like it was water? I was sat on top of a rucksack which contained one change of clothes, some toiletries and a sleeping bag. It was a far cry from lounging on my old comfy three-seater couch in my warm three-bedroomed house. Instead of feeling safe and secure within the four walls of my living room, I felt exposed and horribly conscious of the fact that I was now surrounded by two grey, stony cold walls and a door to a clothes shop that I could not possibly afford to shop in.

I was sat on top of a rucksack which contained one change of clothes, some toiletries and a sleeping bag.

Even though it was around four o'clock in the afternoon, it was a gloomy, dark day. It was raining hard and there were great big puddles of dirty water forming on the pavement in front of me. I was crying just as hard and tears were pouring down my face, landing on the cold, tiled flooring, creating puddles of a different kind. I was cold and wet as I did not have a decent water-proof coat, only a thin summer fleece which had got wet in the rain. I was soaked to the bone, causing me to shiver uncontrollably. Hopefully the alcohol which I was consuming would work its magic and warm me up. My hands had turned a mottled purple and blue colour, underneath the dirt and grime, and I noticed how dirty my nails had become from the lack of washing. I always tried to wash daily, even if it was at a public toilet sink in the middle of town. The trouble was that I never actually felt any cleaner as there was no privacy, because of people constantly walking in and out. I always had to rush and the idea of a strip wash was just too embarrassing.

This day, however, I had no energy left to even think straight, let alone operate on a physical level. I had hit rock bottom before now, but this was the worst I had ever been. My life had spiralled out of control ever since my children were put into the care of my family, leaving me to deal with all the feelings of guilt and self-loathing that had built up inside my head. I had no one to blame but myself for the awful mess my life had become. My ex-partner, who I had been homeless with a year before, had died tragically after suffering a seizure from which he had never recovered. We had been together for three years and I had loved him, despite our destructive relationship, due to drink and drugs. We had had an unpleasant break-up, but after a year apart we had become friends again and made our peace. Now I felt so alone without him and it broke my heart to suddenly be mourning him.

I had hit rock bottom before now, but this was the worst I had ever been.

I looked up as I heard the sound of laughter and saw that there were a couple of kids dressed in matching blue raincoats and yellow wellington boots, jumping and splashing through the ever-deepening puddles. They were being hurried along by their mother who was peering out from under her pink, flowery umbrella. As she noticed me, she quickly averted her eyes. I wondered if she felt pity for me or disgust at this dirty, tramp-like woman sat in a doorway. She shouted at her kids to get a move on and then they all disappeared around a corner.

When you are living on the streets, no one talks to you. You feel shunned and isolated from the rest of society. People look at you but they don't really see you. They look and look away. They walk past quickly. What do they think I am going to do? What are they afraid of? The only people that talk to you are other homeless people and even with them, you have to be careful who you trust. You grow up quick living on the streets. You harden up and you toughen up – except today – I didn't feel very hard or very tough today.

Considering the weather, the street was busier than I expected. I had always enjoyed people-watching and wondering what their lives were like. I used to make up scenarios in my head and try to imagine what job each individual had and whether they were married and what their houses were like. As far as I was concerned they all had their dream homes and grand lifestyles. Now though, I loathed watching these people, who seemed worlds apart from me. I was full of self-hate and pity for my sorry excuse of a life and I felt extremely envious of anyone who had a door to close behind them. My philosophy on life used to be so positive, trying to do good for others and live and let live. I used to see good in people and learn what I could from difficult situations. But all of a sudden my thinking had become twisted and irrational.

But then I saw a familiar, friendly face: my friend Dave with his unmistakable hat and scruffy looking dog, Barney. It filled me with relief to see him. He was my 'Street Dad'. A Street Dad is someone who looks out for you – like a real Dad. And I could talk to Dave about so many things.

'All right love,' he said in a soft, caring voice. He sat down beside me and gave me a cuddle. 'You don't look yourself today. What's up girl?'

'I just feel like ending it all. I can't take another day of this crap,' I said, trying to hold back the tears.

'You know I'm always here if you need me. Do you wanna chat?' he said kindly.

I felt relief flooding over me and I told him how I was feeling. His dog sat down beside me and I stroked him. I started to feel better. Having someone to talk to meant so much. But, he had things to do, and after a while he got up and left, and I was alone again.

After a few long hours, I got up slowly and walked stiffly to the car park where I was to stay the night. As I got there and pushed open the door to the stairwell I was hit with the putrid smell of urine and I quickly covered my nose with my wet sleeve, breathing through my mouth until I got used to it. I unpacked my rucksack, took my sleeping bag out and laid it down on the hard, cold floor. I took off my wet fleece and crawled into the bag's warmth.

As I lay there with my eyes closed I prayed that I would not wake to another day of mental torture.

I could hear someone coughing and spitting in the stairwell below me and then a couple of minutes later I heard the sound of urine splashing against one of the many graffitied walls. It sounded like they were peeing on the same level as me and it echoed round the stairwells for what seemed like minutes. I started to feel scared and wished that I had a companion to protect me. At least when you are a homeless couple you can look out for each other. Being a woman on my own and alone in a dark car park is one of the most scary situations to be in. I felt so vulnerable. As I lay there with my eyes closed I prayed that I would not wake to another day of mental torture. Even if that meant not waking up at all.

Oh how different my life had become compared to the dreams and aspirations of that little girl. How I wished I could be that little girl again.